Jaypee Gold Standard Mini Atlas Series
PHACOEMULSIFICATION

System requirements:

- Operating System—Windows Vista or above
- Web Browser—Google Chrome, Mozilla Firefox, Internet Explorer 9 and above
- Essential plugins—Java and Flash player
  - Facing problems in viewing content—it may be your system does not have Java enabled.
  - If videos do not show up—it may be the system requires Flash player or need to manage flash setting. To learn more about Flash setting, click on the link in the help section.
  - You can test Java and Flash by using the links from the help section of the CD/DVD.

Accompanying DVD-ROM is playable only in Computer and not in DVD player.
CD/DVD has autorun function—it may take few seconds to load on your computer. If it does not work for you, then follow the steps below to access the contents manually:
- Click on my computer
- Select the **CD/DVD** drive and click open/explore—this will show list of files in the **CD/DVD**
- Find and double click file—"launch.html"

For more information about troubleshoot of Autorun click on: (http://support.microsoft.com/kb/330135)

DVD Contents

1. Angle Kappa and Multifocal Glued IOL
2. Intraocular Lens (IOL) Scaffold
3. Lens Coloboma
4. Mature Cataract + Adherent Leucoma + Posterior Synechia
5. No-assistant Technique
6. Pars Plicata Anterior Vitrectomy (PPAV)
7. Subluxated Bag—IOL Complex with Dislocated Ring and Endocapsular Segment

Jaypee Gold Standard Mini Atlas Series
PHACOEMULSIFICATION

Second Edition

Editors

Amar Agarwal MS FRCS FRCOphth
Chairman and Managing Director
Dr Agarwal's Group of Eye Hospitals and Eye Research Center
Chennai, Tamil Nadu, India
Past President
International Society of Refractive Surgery (ISRS)
Secretary General
Indian Intraocular Implant and Refractive Society (IIRSI)

Priya Narang MS
Director
Narang Eye Care and Laser Center
Ahmedabad, Gujarat, India

Foreword
Steven Safran

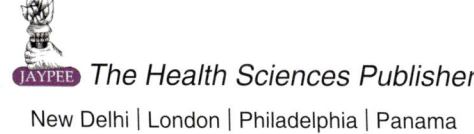

JAYPEE *The Health Sciences Publisher*

New Delhi | London | Philadelphia | Panama

Jaypee Brothers Medical Publishers (P) Ltd.

Headquarters
Jaypee Brothers Medical Publishers (P) Ltd.
4838/24, Ansari Road, Daryaganj
New Delhi 110 002, India
Phone: +91-11-43574357
Fax: +91-11-43574314
E-mail: jaypee@jaypeebrothers.com

Overseas Offices

J.P. Medical Ltd.
83, Victoria Street, London
SW1H 0HW (UK)
Phone: +44-20-3170-8910
Fax: +44(0)-20-3008-6180
E-mail: info@jpmedpub.com

Jaypee-Highlights Medical Publishers Inc.
City of Knowledge, Bld. 237, Clayton
Panama City, Panama
Phone: +1 507-301-0496
Fax: +1 507-301-0499
E-mail: cservice@jphmedical.com

Jaypee Medical Inc.
The Bourse
111, South Independence Mall East
Suite 835, Philadelphia, PA 19106, USA
Phone: +1 267-519-9789
E-mail: jpmed.us@gmail.com

Jaypee Brothers Medical Publishers (P) Ltd.
17/1-B, Babar Road, Block-B, Shaymali
Mohammadpur, Dhaka-1207
Bangladesh
Mobile: +08801912003485
E-mail: jaypeedhaka@gmail.com

Jaypee Brothers Medical Publishers (P) Ltd.
Bhotahity, Kathmandu, Nepal
Phone: +977-9741283608
E-mail: kathmandu@jaypeebrothers.com

Website: www.jaypeebrothers.com
Website: www.jaypeedigital.com

© 2015, Jaypee Brothers Medical Publishers

The views and opinions expressed in this book are solely those of the original contributor(s)/author(s) and do not necessarily represent those of editor(s) of the book.

All rights reserved. No part of this publication and DVD-ROM may be reproduced, stored or transmitted in any form or by any means, electronic, mechanical, photocopying, recording or otherwise, without the prior permission in writing of the publishers

All brand names and product names used in this book are trade names, service marks, trademarks or registered trademarks of their respective owners. The publisher is not associated with any product or vendor mentioned in this book.

Medical knowledge and practice change constantly. This book is designed to provide accurate, authoritative information about the subject matter in question. However, readers are advised to check the most current information available on procedures included and check information from the manufacturer of each product to be administered, to verify the recommended dose, formula, method and duration of administration, adverse effects and contraindications. It is the responsibility of the practitioner to take all appropriate safety precautions. Neither the publisher nor the author(s)/editor(s) assume any liability for any injury and/or damage to persons or property arising from or related to use of material in this book.

This book is sold on the understanding that the publisher is not engaged in providing professional medical services. If such advice or services are required, the services of a competent medical professional should be sought.

Every effort has been made where necessary to contact holders of copyright to obtain permission to reproduce copyright material. If any have been inadvertently overlooked, the publisher will be pleased to make the necessary arrangements at the first opportunity.

Inquiries for bulk sales may be solicited at: jaypee@jaypeebrothers.com

Jaypee Gold Standard Mini Atlas Series: Phacoemulsification

First Edition: 2007
Second Edition: **2015**

ISBN: 978-93-5152-784-8

Printed at : Samrat Offset Pvt. Ltd.

Dedicated to

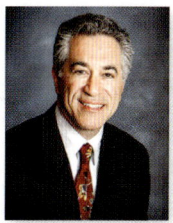

Donald Serafano

Foreword to the Second Edition

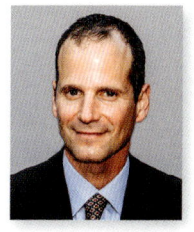

The first time I met Dr Amar Agarwal, I was presenting at the 2011 American Society of Cataract and Refractive Surgery (ASCRS): Complications and Challenging Cases in Cataract Surgery Video Symposium, where there was an award for the best case of session. I presented second to the last, had a very challenging and compelling case, and gave what I thought was a pretty solid presentation; so I felt pretty good about my chances to win. This feeling lasted about 30 seconds into the following and final presentation, which was given by Dr Amar Agarwal. Of course, I had known of Dr Amar Agarwal because of his work, but I had never had the opportunity to meet him personally. He took the podium, and with his surprisingly booming voice, self-effacing manner coupled with his wonderful sense of humor, had the audience transfixed within a few moments. He proceeded to take us all through a whirlwind journey of a case, where every possible complication, one can think of, occurred and was dealt with by a surgeon, who had unparalleled daring skill, experience and the willingness to honestly share the trials and tribulations of eye surgery, as it was the most challenging moment. Of course, Dr Amar Agarwal won the best case of session. The same thing happened in 2013 at the ASCRS video symposium, I attended, where again, he presented the last and just blew everyone away with his skill, humor and humble manner in a presentation for the ages. I have learned that presenting a case right before Dr Amar Agarwal takes the podium, is a bit such as performing at the Grammy's right before Beyoncé does. Good luck with that.

Since 2011, I was fortunate to become friend with Dr Amar Agarwal and learn more personally from his incredible wealth of experience. He has a rare level of energy and excitement for what he does; and when he shares his knowledge, it is with a unique level of enthusiasm and his trademark humble honesty that makes him so approachable. I do not know what time it is in Chennai, Tamil Nadu, India, when I text or e-mail from New Jersey with a question about a difficult case but I do know that Amar Agarwal always replies within seconds. When I recently presented a group of colleagues with a challenging case via e-mail asking for their thoughts and comments to be published in an article, I was writing, Amar Agarwal was the first to respond with a detailed, well-thought out, publishable response within less than an hour. Now I know that it is the middle of the night for him so I have to wonder... does he sleep? Perhaps, not, because, if you look at all of his contribution to our profession, his travel schedule, the meetings all over the world, he presents at and the incredible caseload, he manages as a surgeon, you begin to suspect that perhaps he is working while the rest of us are not.

Foreword to the Second Edition

He has given us advances in many areas of ophthalmic surgery and this is no doubt because he has skill and experience that transcends so many subspecialties. As a cataract surgeon with training in vitreoretinal surgery, he has been able to synthesize ideas and techniques from both disciplines. This has given us advances in intraocular lens fixation in the absence of capsular support that has revolutionized how we approach our aphakic and dislocated intraocular lens (IOL) patients. His "glued in" intraocular lens method and the use of an IOL scaffold to complete cases in the absence of capsular support has revolutionized how we approach our complicated cases. He has brought us many advances in phacoemulsification methods through the decades, which have been chronicled in his many articles and textbooks and has contributed recently a new method in endothelial keratoplasty as well. Surgeons from all over the world come to visit Dr Amar Agarwal and learn from him personally at his eye hospital in Chennai, when he is not traveling or doing live surgery to teach "on the road". I have learned to pick his brain when I see him in person at meetings and to save my toughest cases to present to him when I have the opportunity to corner him between his running from one place to the next. Of course, I could just text him because I know he will respond as he always does, in a matter of seconds without fail no matter what time, it is but it is so much more fun to see the light in his eyes in person as he enthusiastically shares his experience.

In the book he shares some of his incredible experiences in surgical steps and complication management during modern cataract surgery. The book will provide something that both the novice and most gifted, and experienced surgeons can expect to gain new insight and knowledge. He is a force of nature that happens to be an ophthalmologist and we are fortunate to have his voice amongst us.

Steven Safran MD
Consultant
Capital Health System
New Jersey Surgery Center
Robert Wood Johnson University Hospital
Hamilton, USA

Foreword to the First Edition

Probably no technique in the history of Ophthalmology has stirred as much interest and literature as phacoemulsification has. This is caused, not only by the frequency of the disease it treats, but also because of the ever-evolving and demanding technique and technology.

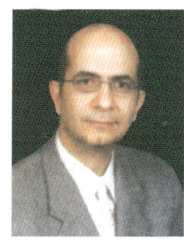

This Mini Atlas on Phacoemulsification we have in our hands offers us a concise, well-illustrated and demonstrative approach to intricacies of the phaco world. With so many photographs and illustrations, the Mini Atlas is an easily accessible and navigable data source.

It starts with a section on basics of phaco and the simple, yet very helpful concept of gas-forced infusion forwarded by Sunita Agarwal a few years ago, going through other steps of the phaco technique. A section on tough cases like subluxated nuclei then follows.

Complications and nightmares do face even the most experienced surgeon, and on these, thanks to the phenomenal number of cases done and taught at the Agarwal Hospitals, a special section is dedicated.

We all remember the debate between the classical extracapsular and phaco surgeons in the mid-late 1980s, and whether it was worthy to make a 3.2 mm incision to be widened later to implant then only available 6 mm diameter lens. We all knew the 3.2 mm incision would eventually win, and so it did! For the past few years, we are facing a similar (smaller) debate with the introduction of phaconit by Dr Agarwal which was popularized as microphaco, bimanual phaco, or microincision cataract surgery (MICS). Dr Agarwal is still going down the millimeter scale and is now presenting phaco through a 0.7 mm tip. Advances in IOL manufacturing and technology will no doubt help these surgical achievements more and more. Will the day come when we look back at the horribly large 3.2 mm incision?

Once again, Dr Amar Agarwal presents us with a fine addition to the library of Ophthalmology, which is a very helpful companion for all surgeons aspiring to improve their surgical results using the latest techniques available.

Ahmad K Khalil MD PhD
Associate Professor of Ophthalmology
National Research Institute of Ophthalmology
Board Member and Treasurer
Egyptian Society for Cataract and Corneal Diseases
Office Bearer, Egyptian Society of the Glaucomas
Office: Saridar Clinic Tower
92 Tahrir St. Dokki, Cairo, Egypt
www.eyecairo.net

Preface to the Second Edition

Jaypee Gold Standard Mini Atlas Series: Phacoemulsification is now in its second edition, and the previous edition has corresponded to a different phase in the way the graphics and pictures were displayed all over the book. In order to understand what it means to successfully understand the various clinical scenarios encountered in practice the surgical skills and an understanding of the key elements is critical to achieving the optimum visual outcome. The book has been written to provide a framework for learning these necessary skills in a way that emphasizes the uniqueness of each clinical condition. Following the images is the text that emphasizes and describes the essence of the clinical condition and various ways to deal with it effectively.

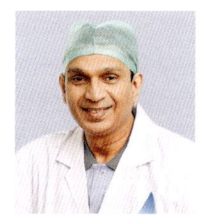

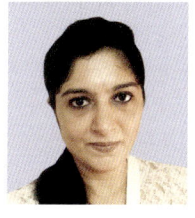

The main goal of writing the book was to embark upon the features of accuracy and a structured approach that results from many years of facilitating, researching and teaching. The book places not only a clear emphasis on teaching skills first but also ensures that those skills are based on rigorous and current research. We hope that the book sets a framework that allows the readers to gain new information and current concepts in surgical practice into a larger context.

Jaypee Gold Standard Mini Atlas Series: Phacoemulsification speaks of fundamental component of an atlas that displays images of phacoemulsification surgery in varied situations. The book has four sections and a DVD with videos showcasing the surgical aspects of handling numerous clinical conditions related to phacoemulsification and its complications. We hope that the book benefits all the readers so that the knowledge is transferred in dealing successfully with our patients to enhance the visual outcomes.

Amar Agarwal
Priya Narang

Preface to the First Edition

Cataract surgery has become extremely delicate. The reason is as we go smaller and smaller moving from the extracapsular cataract extraction (ECCE) to phaco to microphakonit the surgery gets more demanding. That is the reason why this book has been written. The idea is basically to teach everyone the intricacies of the surgical techniques.

The book is a small book so that it can be kept in the operation theater or carried in the hand. When one is starting a tough case, the book can be read easily so that the difficulty of the case can be easily conquered. There are lots of figures also in the book so that one can understand the concept easily.

We hope the book will help you master the surgery in a faster and better way. We would like to thank Shri Jitendar P Vij (Group Chairman) of M/s Jaypee Brothers Medical Publishers (P) Ltd, New Delhi, India and the others of Jaypee to help us bring out the book.

Sunita Agarwal
Athiya Agarwal
Amar Agarwal

Contents

Section 1 PHACO BASICS
Amar Agarwal, Priya Narang

- Diagrammatic Representation of the Connection of Air Pump to the Infusion Bottle — 2
- Internal Gas Forced Infusion — 4
- Viscoelastic being Injected with a 26 G Needle Attached to a 1 mL Syringe — 6
- Framing a Clear Corneal Incision — 8
  - Location of the Incision *9*
  - Size of the Incision *9*
  - Plane of the Incision *10*
- Capsulorhexis being done with a Bent 26 Gauge Needle — 11
- Capsulorhexis Flap — 12
- Vertical Chop — 15
- Chopping the Nuclear Hemisegments — 17
- Pull out Nuclear Fragments from Bag and Emulsify — 19
- Bi-manual Cortical Aspiration — 20

Section 2 CHALLENGING CASES
Amar Agarwal, Priya Narang

- Pseudoexfoliation — 24
- Deposition of Fluffy Amorphous Material Around the Pupil in Pseudoexfoliation — 25
- Pigment Deposition on Anterior Capsule — 27

xviii | Phacoemulsification

- Posterior Synechia — 28
- Posterior Polar Cataract — 30
- Trypan Blue Enhanced Capsulorhexis being Performed in a Miotic, Fibrotic Pupil — 32
  - Surgical Tips *33*
- Subluxation of the Lens and its Management — 37
- Modified Cionni's Capsular Tension Ring — 39
- Lenticular Coloboma — 41
- Iris Coloboma — 43
- Soemmering Ring — 44
- Posterior Lenticonus — 46

Section 3 COMPLICATIONS
Amar Agarwal, Priya Narang

- Sleeveless Phacotip Assisted Levitation of Dropped Nucleus (SPAL) Technique—Step 1 — 50
- Spal Technique—Step 2 — 53
- Dropped Nucleus Lying on the Retina — 54
  - Managing the Anterior Chamber Opacities and Herniated Vitreous *55*
  - Posterior Vitrectomy and Phacofragmentation *56*
- Insulating the Retina with Perfluorocarbon — 59
- Principle of an Ophthalmic Endoscopic System — 60
- Removal of Entire Hard Lens Fragment with Perfluorocarbon — 64

- Management of Lens Coloboma with Glued IOL — 69
- Dislocated IOL on the Retina — 72
    - Sleeveless Extrusion Cannula for Levitation of Dropped IOL *72*
    - Surgical Technique *73*
    - Perfluorocarbon Liquids *76*
- 25-G Chang Passive-Action IOL Forceps — 78
- Temporary Haptic Externalization — 80
- Removal of a Plate Haptic IOL — 84
- Management of Eyes with two Intraocular Implants — 87
- Endophthalmitis: Methods of Collecting Specimens — 90
    - Clinical Features *91*
    - Organisms Associated with Acute Postoperative Endophthalmitis *93*
    - Delayed-onset Endophthalmitis *94*
    - Propionibacterium Endophthalmitis *94*
    - Diagnostic Workup and Microbiological Studies *96*
    - Techniques of Specimen Collection *97*
- Endophthalmitis (Anterior Chamber Washout before Vitrectomy) — 99
    - Antimicrobial Therapy *100*
    - Corticosteroid Therapy *103*
    - Vitrectomy *104*
- Cystoid Macular Edema — 107
    - Macular Edema *108*
    - Cystoid Macular Edema *108*
    - Cme and Aciol—Possible Pathophysiology *112*
    - Clinical Appearance of CME *113*

Macular Function Tests
in Cystoid Macular Edema *116*

- Optical Coherence Tomography in CME   116
  Sequela of CME: Post-CME Lamellar Hole *117*
  Prophylactic Treatment *118*
  Therapy for Established CME *119*

- Glued IOL   123
- Glued IOL (Continued)   125
- Traumatic Iridodialysis   127
- Boston Keratoprosthesis (KPro)   129
- Decentration of the Capsular Bag and IOL   131
- IOL Scaffold   132
- Glued IOL Scaffold   134
- Pre-Descemet's Endothelial Keratyoplasty with Glued IOL   137
  Surgical Considerations
  for Combined Procedure *140*
  Surgical Technique *140*
- Preoperative and Postoperative Image of Patient of PDEK with Glued IOL   142
  Refractive Concern *144*

Section 4 MICROINCISION CATARACT SURGERY (PHAKONIT AND MICROPHAKONIT)

Amar Agarwal, Priya Narang

- Clear Corneal Incision Made with a Special Knife (MST, USA)   146
- Capsulorhexis Initiated with a Needle   148

- MST Rhexis Forceps used to Perform the Rhexis in a Mature Cataract — 150
- Designs of Agarwal Irrigating Choppers — 151
- Phakonit Irrigating Chopper and Phako Probe without the Sleeve Inside the Eye — 152
- Phakonit being done — 154
- Bimanual Irrigation Aspiration Completed — 155
- Soft Tip Irrigation-aspiration from MST, USA — 156
- Thinoptx Roller Cum Injector Inserting the IOL in the Capsular Bag — 157
- Comparison between Phaco Foldable IOL and Phakonit Thinoptx IOL — 158
- Microphakonit — 160
- Microphakonit Completed. The Nucleus has been Removed — 162
- Bimanual Irrigation-aspiration with the 0.7 mm Set — 164
- Bimanual Irrigation-aspiration Completed — 165

Index — *167*

SECTION 1

Phaco Basics

Amar Agarwal
Priya Narang

DIAGRAMMATIC REPRESENTATION OF THE CONNECTION OF AIR PUMP TO THE INFUSION BOTTLE

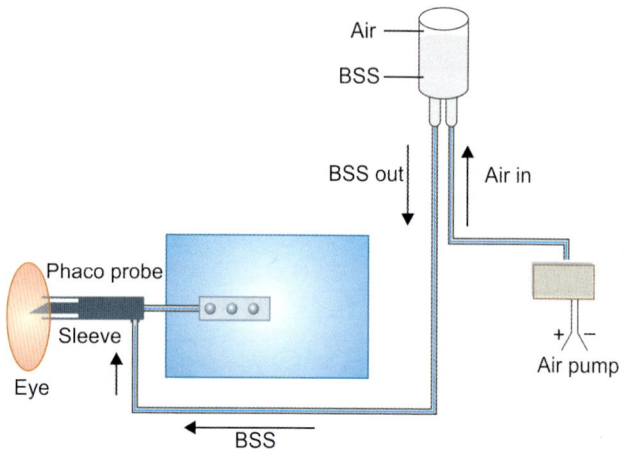

Fig. 1.1 Diagrammatic representation of the connection of air pump to the infusion bottle

Abbreviation: BSS; Balanced salt solution

The problem encountered in bimanual phaco/phakonit was the destabilization of the anterior chamber during surgery. It was solved to a certain extent by using an 18 gauge irrigating chopper. Dr Sunita Agarwal suggested the use of an antichamber collapser, which injects air into the infusion bottle (Fig. 1.1). This helps to push more fluid into the eye through the irrigating chopper and also prevent surge. This allowed the usage of a 20 gauge or 21 gauge irrigating chopper and also solved the issue of destabilization of the anterior chamber during surgery. In microphakonit surgery, due to gas forced infusion, it was possible to remove cataracts with a 0.7 mm irrigating chopper. Subsequently, this system was employed in all the coaxial phacoemulsification cases done at our center to prevent complications like posterior capsular rupture and corneal damage.

The concept of employing air pump originated from the use of a locally manufactured automated device used in fish tanks (aquariums) to supply oxygen, which was utilized to forcefully pump air into the irrigation bottle. It has an electromagnetic motor which moves a lever attached to a collapsible rubber cap. There is an inlet with a valve, which sucks in atmospheric air as the cap expands. On collapsing, the valve closes and the air is pushed into an intravenous (IV) line connected to the infusion bottle. The lever vibrates at a frequency of approximately 10 oscillations per second. The electromagnetic motor is weak enough to stop once the pressure in the closed system (i.e. the anterior chamber) reaches about 50 mm of Hg. The rubber cap ceases to expand at this pressure level. A micropore air filter is used between the air pump and the infusion bottle so that the air pumped into the bottle is clean of particulate matter.

This was the origin of the idea of 'Forced gas infusion' that is now employed in almost all the top end phaco machines to maintain the chamber stability.

INTERNAL GAS FORCED INFUSION

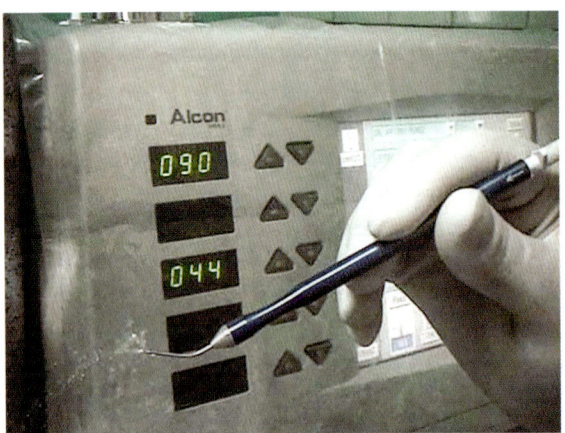

Fig. 1.2 Internal gas forced infusion
(*Courtesy:* Arturo Pérez Arteaga, Mexico)

Arturo Pérez-Arteaga from Mexico started internal gas forced infusion. The anterior vented gas forced infusion system (AVGFI) of the accurus surgical system (Fig. 1.2) creates a positive infusion pressure inside the eye; it was designed by the Alcon engineers to control the intraocular pressure (IOP) during the anterior and posterior segment surgery. It consists of an air pump and a regulator which are inside the machine that push the air inside the bottle of intraocular solution which in return actively pushes the fluid inside the eye without the need to raise or lower the bottle height. The control of the air pump is digitally integrated in the Accurus panel; it can also be controlled via the remote. The footswitch can be preset with the minimal and maximum of desired fluid inside the eye and it almost reaches this value directly with a single tap on the footswitch. Arturo Pérez-Arteaga recommends presetting the infusion pump at 100 to 110 mm of Hg. It is a strong irrigation force to perform a microincision phaco and this parameter is preset in the panel as well as in the foot switch as the minimal irrigation. It is recommended to preset the maximum irrigation force at 130 to 140 mm of Hg in the foot pedal, so if a surge ever occurs during the procedure the surgeon can increase the irrigation force by the simple touch of the footswitch to the right. With the AVGFI the surgeon has the capability to increase these values to a higher level if needed.

VISCOELASTIC BEING INJECTED WITH A 26 G NEEDLE ATTACHED TO A 1 mL SYRINGE

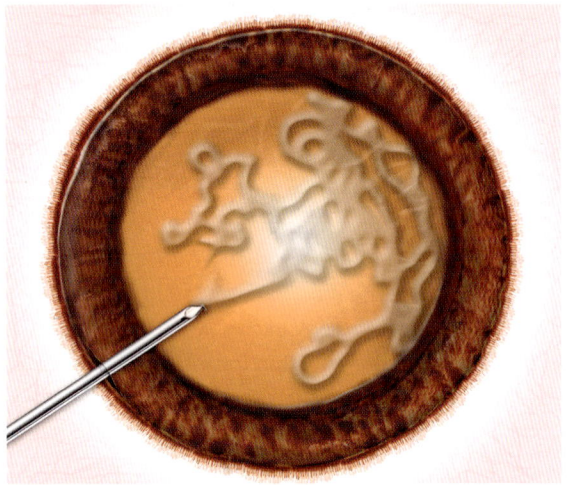

Fig. 1.3 Viscoelastic being injected from the side port incision. This makes the eye taut and facilitates better fashioning of the valvular corneal tunnel

Before the cataract surgery is begun, the authors recommend distending the eye with viscoelastic. This can be achieved by attaching a 26 G needle to a 1 mL syringe that is laden with viscoelastic. The surgeon enters the eye at the site of the future sideport incision and injects viscoelastic (Fig. 1.3). This makes the eye taut and helps the surgeon to frame a better valvular corneal section.

This step is especially beneficial in 'Topical' as well as 'No anesthesia' cataract surgery. On 13th June 1998 at Ahmedabad, India the first 'No. anesthesia' cataract surgery was done by Dr Amar Agarwal as a live surgery at the Phaco and Refractive Surgery conference that opened up various new concepts in the arena of cataract surgery. This is the most important step as it gives an entry into the eye through which a straight rod can be passed to stabilize the eye during the entire course of surgery.

Phacoemulsification

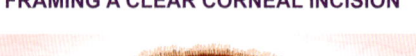

FRAMING A CLEAR CORNEAL INCISION

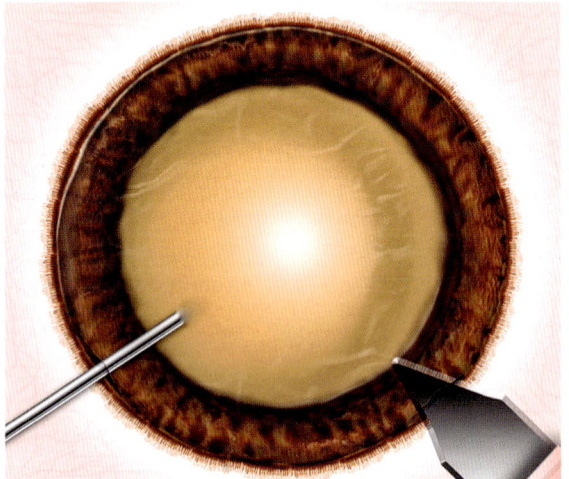

Fig. 1.4 Corneal tunnel being made with the keratome and a globe stabilization rod is introduced from the sideport incision.
Note: A straight stabilization rod in the left hand to stabilize the globe while the right hand performs the clear corneal incision

Framing a clear corneal incision is a very important step of phacoemulsification surgery. The location of the incision, length, thickness, configuration play a very important role in the outcome of the surgery.

The corneal incision is framed with a keratome (Fig. 1.4) that may be either a diamond blade or a stainless steel disposable blade. They are available in different sizes, shapes and bevels.

LOCATION OF THE INCISION

The location of the incision can be chosen depending on the axis of the astigmatism. When the incision is framed, it tends to cause flattening in the meridian of the incision and steepening in the perpendicular axis. The degree of astigmatism depends on the distance of the incision from the center of the cornea, the size of the incision, and its shape. Astigmatism is inversely proportional to the incision's distance from the limbus and directly proportional to the cube of the incision's length.

Currently, surgeons prefer to create a temporal incision rather than superior. However, some surgeons prefer to place the incision on the steep meridian and therefore they operate along the concerned meridian.

SIZE OF THE INCISION

Size of the incision refers to the width and length of the wound. The width of the incision is determined by gauge or thickness of phaco needle and the IOL design. It varies in MICS (micro-incision cataract surgery) and routine cataract surgery. The advantage of a smaller incision is reduced astigmatic effect, and those shorter than 3 mm are considered to be astigmatically neutral. The most stable wound configuration is square, with the length of the tunnel as long as the width of the incision.

PLANE OF THE INCISION

The plane of the incision can be uniplanar, biplanar or triplanar.

Uniplanar incisions are practiced currently. The keratome is entered into the eye in a single horizontal beveled movement so as enter into the anterior chamber.

Biplanar wounds have a larger surface area than uniplanar ones, and may be more stable. The initial partial-thickness groove is made perpendicular to the cornea followed by a beveled entry into the anterior chamber.

Triplanar incisions (perpendicular-beveled-perpendicular) consist of an internal corneal lip created by redirecting the keratome tip ("dimple down" maneuver followed by reorienting the keratome parallel to the iris). This functions as a one-way valve and produces a self-sealing, water tight wound when made correctly. If, however, the keratome is angled downward, upward, or tilted sideways while incising Descemet's membrane, then instead of being straight, the shape of the internal incision will be an arrowhead, V, or S, respectively, and the internal valve function may be compromised.

CAPSULORHEXIS BEING DONE WITH A BENT 26 GAUGE NEEDLE

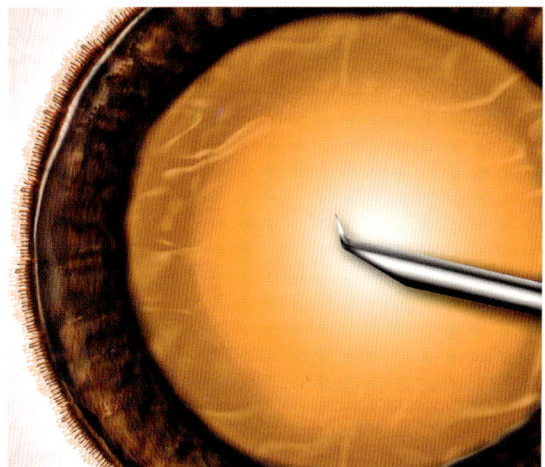

Fig. 1.5 The tip of a 26 G needle is bent for the capsulorhexis

Capsulorhexis is performed either with a 26 G (Fig. 1.5) needle or with a capsulorhexis forceps through the corneal incision and the choice depends entirely on the surgeon's preference. In pediatric and young patients, it is preferable to do capsulorhexis with a forceps as it offers better control over the edges of the flap created. In young patients, the surgeon should intend to create a capsulorhexis of around 5 mm initially as it often tends to run in the periphery due to increased posterior pressure and elasticity of the capsule.

CAPSULORHEXIS FLAP

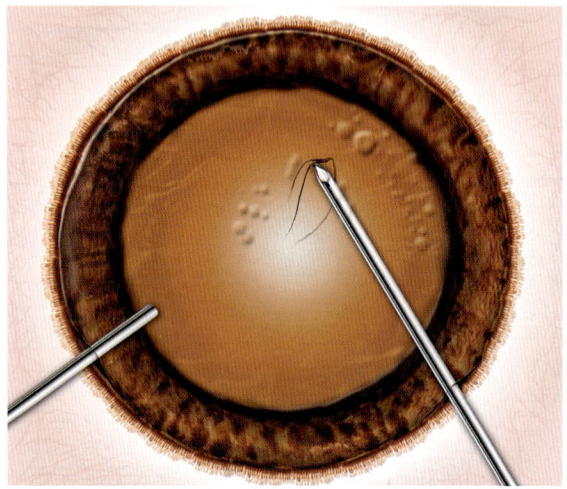

Fig. 1.6 Capsulorhexis initiated with a bent 26 G needle

While performing the capsulorhexis, it is important to start the capsulorhexis from the center (Fig. 1.6) and move the needle to the right and then downward. This is important, as the concepts have changed and it is better to remember it as superior, inferior, right or left. If the surgeon happens to start the capsulorhexis from the center and move towards the left then the weakest point of the capsulorhexis is generally where it ends. In other words, the point where the surgeon tends to lose

Phaco Basics

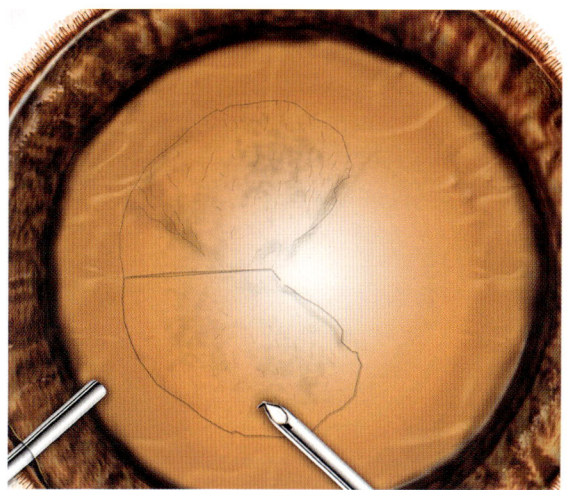

Fig. 1.7 Capsulorhexis in process and the anterior capsular flap is seen

the capsulorhexis is near its completion. So the surgeon will have an incomplete capsulorhexis on the left-hand side either inferiorly or superiorly. As, the phaco probe is always moved down and to the left so with every stroke of movement with the phaco probe the rhexis gets extended posteriorly creating a posterior capsular rupture. Alternatively, if the surgeon performs the rhexis from the center and move to the right and pushes the flap inferiorly (Fig. 1.7) then in a case of incomplete rhexis it will be near the end of the rhexis and it will be located superiorly and to the right. Any incomplete rhexis can extend and create a posterior capsular tear but in the latter scenario, the chances of survival are better. This is because we are moving the phaco probe down and to the left, but the rhexis is incomplete up and to the right.

VERTICAL CHOP

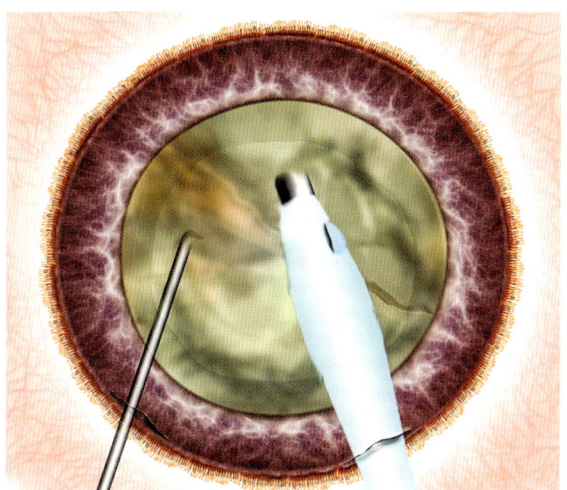

Fig. 1.8 Vertical chop being performed and the nucleus is divided into two halves

For the chop technique, the authors tend to use Agarwal chopper that is a sharp chopper with sharp cutting edge and a sharp point (Fig. 1.8). It offers an advantage that the surgeon can work and chop the nucleus in the center itself without the need of going into the periphery of the nucleus. This helps especially in cases with small pupil as the chopper always remain within the confines of the rhexis margin.

The phaco tip is embedded slightly superior to the center of the nucleus and the ultrasound energy is applied so that the tip gets embedded at the center of the nucleus. The direction of the phaco probe should be obliquely downwards toward the vitreous and not horizontally towards the iris. The settings of the phaco machine depend on the density of the cataract. For the chopping technique, it is preferable to use a zero or a 15° phaco tip as it gets embedded in the nucleus very well and helps in achieving better chops.

Once the tip is embedded, the surgeon goes to foot pedal position 2 so that only suction is being used. The nucleus is slightly lifted so as not to apply any inadvertent pressure on the posterior capsule during the process of chopping. The surgeon then cuts the nucleus with the chopper in a straight downward motion and then moves the chopper to the left when the center of the nucleus is reached. In other words, the left hand moves the chopper like a laterally reversed 'L'. This creates a crack and the nucleus gets split into two pieces.

CHOPPING THE NUCLEAR HEMISEGMENTS

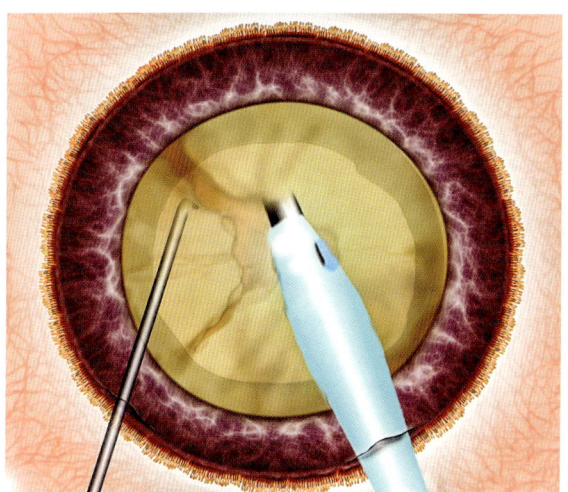

Fig. 1.9 Further chops created in the heminucleus

As two halves of the nucleus is attained, the surgeon rotates the nucleus and tries to place the phaco probe into one half of the nucleus with the direction of the probe being horizontal as the aim is to shelf the nucleus (Fig. 1.9).

As described above, create at least 3 chops in one half of the nucleus. Similarly, after rotation 3 halves are attained in the remaining part of the nucleus. Thus, 6 quadrants or pie-shaped fragments are achieved at the end of chopping procedure. The settings at this stage are 50% phaco power, 24 mL/minute flow rate and 101 mm of Hg suction.

Remember 5 words protocol: Embed, Pull, Chop, Split and Release.

PULL OUT NUCLEAR FRAGMENTS FROM BAG AND EMULSIFY

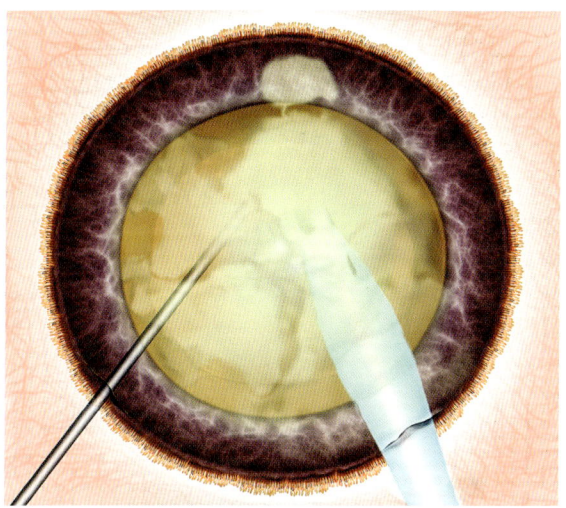

Fig. 1.10 Nuclear fragments being pulled out from the bag and subsequent emulsification being performed

Once all the pieces have been chopped, pull out each piece one by one and in pulse phaco mode aspirate the pieces at the level of the iris (Fig. 1.10). Do not work in the bag unless the cornea is pre-operatively bad or the patient is very elderly. The setting at this stage can be phaco power 30–50 %, flow rate 24 mL and suction 101 mm of Hg.

BI-MANUAL CORTICAL ASPIRATION

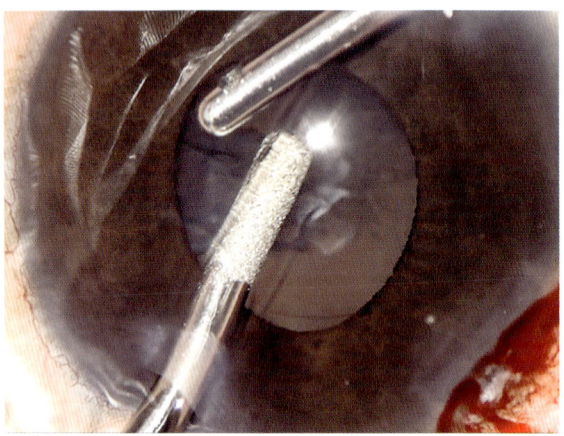

Fig. 1.11 Bi-manual cortical aspiration being performed

Cortical washing is a very important aspect of phaco surgery that can be accomplished either with a coaxial or a bimanual probe (Fig. 1.11). Removal of the subincisional cortex is the most tricky part of the procedure that is better accomplished with a bimanual probe as it facilitates the surgeon to switch the probe between the two sideport incisions created for the same and helps in better maneuverability. Special 'J' shaped I/A probe is alsoavailable for the sub incisional aspiration of cortical material.

At the completion of the procedure, a foldable IOL is loaded and is injected into the eye. Stromal hydration is done to seal the corneal incisions by injecting BSS inside the lips of the clear corneal incision. This creates water tight wound and the incisions are sealed better.

SECTION 2

Challenging Cases

Amar Agarwal
Priya Narang

PSEUDOEXFOLIATION

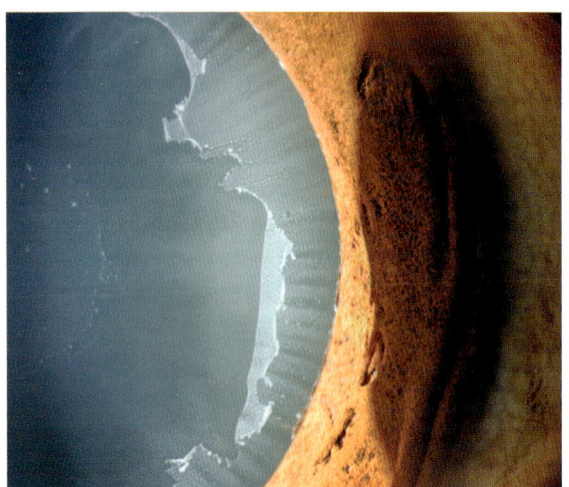

Fig. 2.1 Characteristic delamination of the anterior capsule in pseudoexfoliation

Pseudoexfoliation as a term differentiates itself from true exfoliation that was originally seen in glassblowers due to exposure to infra-red rays leading to delamination of the anterior capsule. Pseudoexfoliation syndrome (PXS) is a systemic condition with ocular manifestations wherein the pseudoexfoliation material deposits on various structures of the anterior segment.

The image demonstrates the characteristic peeling or delamination of the anterior capsule (Fig. 2.1).

DEPOSITION OF FLUFFY AMORPHOUS MATERIAL AROUND THE PUPIL IN PSEUDOEXFOLIATION

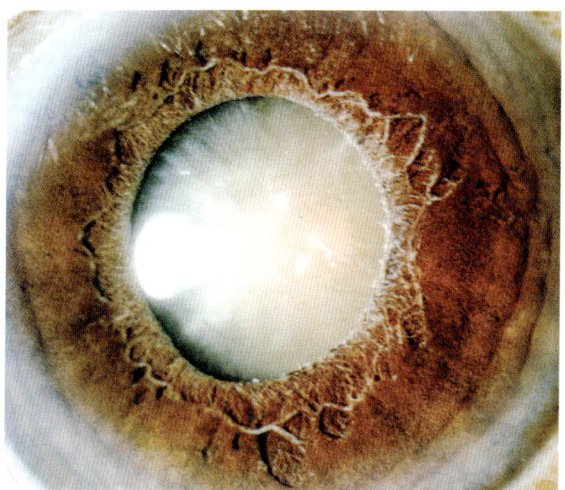

Fig. 2.2 An eye with pseudoexfoliation syndrome.
Note: Fluffy deposits along the pupillary border and a non-dilating pupil with patches of iris depigmentation

The image demonstrates the deposition of fluffy dandruff like structure along the pupillary margin with a non-dilating pupil associated with mature cataract (Fig. 2.2). The characteristic patches of iris depigmentation are seen which in later stages often lead to trans-illumination defects.

In advanced cases, the deposition of fluffy material is also seen on lens zonules and on the trabecular meshwork. This leads to secondary open-angle glaucoma, phacodonesis or lens subluxation caused by zonular dehiscence.

Loss of lens zonular support makes intraocular surgeries challenging with the potential for vitreous loss, lens subluxation, or even lens dislocation into the vitreous cavity.

PIGMENT DEPOSITION ON ANTERIOR CAPSULE

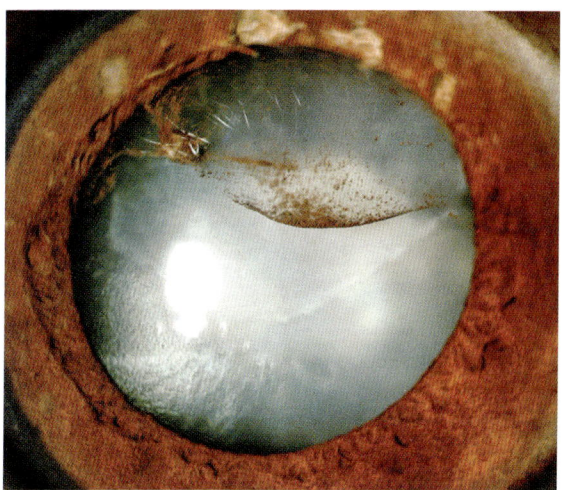

Fig. 2.3 Pigment dispersion on the anterior capsule of the lens

Pigment dispersion may be associated with conditions in which pigment epithelium or uveal melanocytes are injured, such as uveitis, secondary glaucoma or uveal melanoma. The dispersed pigment is presumed to be iris pigment epithelium mechanically rubbed off by contact with lens zonular fibers. There can be pigmentation of the lens (Fig. 2.3), trabecular meshwork or pars plana. The pigmentation may precede glaucoma by as much as 20 years. Pigmentation is often seen after dilation of the eye with cycloplegic drugs in a case of posterior synechiae.

POSTERIOR SYNECHIA

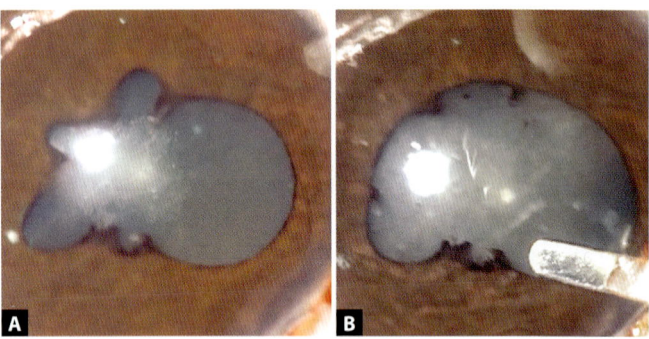

Figs 2.4A and B Posterior synechia in anterior uveitis. (A) Adhesions are present between the posterior surface of iris and the anterior capsule of the lens; (B) Adhesions being released with the help of a blunt iris spatula to facilitate the subsequent dilation of pupil and to avoid damage to the anterior capsular surface

A: The image depicts the presence of posterior synechias on the anterior capsule (Fig. 2.4A). This is usually a sign of previous episode of inflammatory insult. They are often seen in acute anterior uveitis and chronic posterior uveitis. In very extreme cases, it may be associated with angle closure glaucoma due to anterior bowing of the peripheral iris (iris bombè) especially when 360-degree adhesion (seclusio pupillae) occurs.

B: The treatment is initiated with cycloplegic drops and often atropine acts as a wonder drug in such cases. When such cases are associated with cataract, synechiolysis has to be done. After inflating the eye with viscoelastic, an iris spatula is passed beneath the synechias and an attempt is made to break them by a sweeping movement parallel to the plane of the iris (Fig. 2.4B). If the adhesions fail to break then a scissor can be used to cut them and iris hooks can be employed to dilate the pupil and perform the surgery.

POSTERIOR POLAR CATARACT

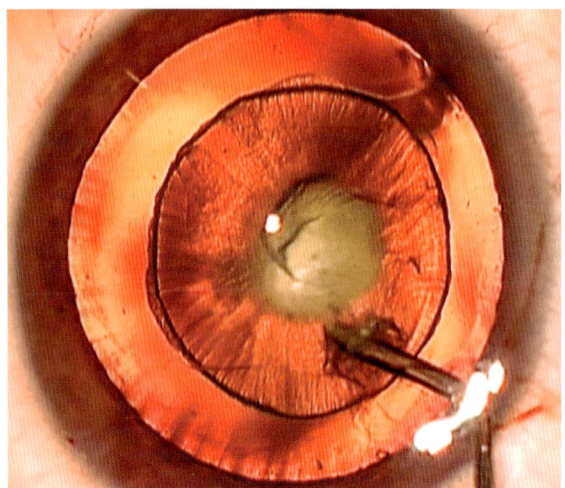

Fig. 2.5 Hydrodelineation being performed in a posterior polar cataract

Posterior polar cataract (PPC) is a clinically distinctive entity consisting of a dense white, well demarcated, disk-shaped opacity located in the posterior cortex or subcapsular region. Two types of PPC have been described in literature: stationary and progressive. The bull's eye appearance is pathognomonic of posterior polar cataracts.

Corticocleaving hydrodissection can lead to hydraulic rupture and should be avoided. It would be logical to perform hydrodelineation to create a mechanical cushion of epinucleus. It is critical that the hydrodelineation needle be inserted into a plane away from the height of the polar cataract (Fig. 2.5) so that when a wave front is created, the posterior capsule is not ruptured. At times the classical appearance suggestive of a defect is observed in the posterior cortex, but the posterior capsule remains intact. This is known as a 'pseudohole'.

TRYPAN BLUE ENHANCED CAPSULORHEXIS BEING PERFORMED IN A MIOTIC, FIBROTIC PUPIL

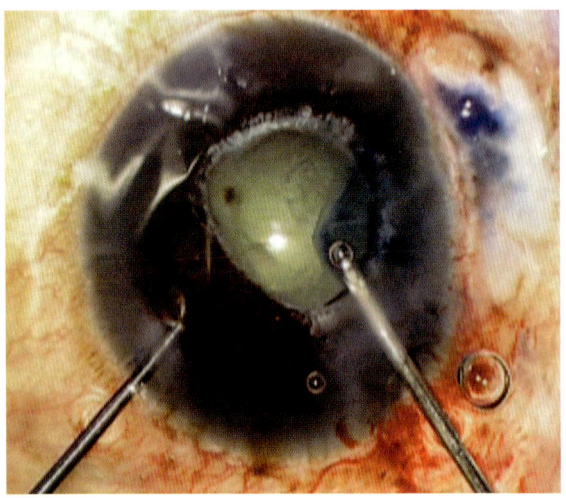

Fig. 2.6 Trypan blue staining of the anterior capsule followed by capsulorhexis in a miotic and fibrotic pupil

Trypan blue enhances the visualization of the anterior capsule (Fig. 2.6) especially in a case of mature and hypermature cataract. Miotic pupil adds to the difficulties experienced by a surgeon in an already mature cataract. Iris hooks or other pupil size enhancing devices can ease the procedure to a great extent.

SURGICAL TIPS

- In cases with small pupil, the corneal incision must be made anteriorly to avoid the risk of iris prolapse with posterior corneal incisions.
- Capsular dyes such as indocyanine green (ICG) or trypan blue (preferred) should be injected under the iris to aid in making the rhexis as well as to visualize the capsule as the pupil later enlarges.
- Hydrodissection should be gentle as an excessive fluid wave can cause iris prolapse.
- A retentive viscoelastic such as Healon 5 should be used as it pressurizes the anterior chamber. As the intraocular pressure (IOP) increases, the viscoelastic remains in the eye and pushes down on the lens-iris diaphragm, thus mechanically enlarging the pupil. A cohesive type of viscoelastic is not as effective as it evacuates easily from the eye when IOP increases.
- Mini-sphincterotomies or the bimanual stretching technique of Luther Fry work well with fibrotic pupils such as those in patients on chronic miotic therapy. They are not as effective when the iris is elastic and floppy because the sphincter does not readily tear and the iris snaps back following stretching.
- A Sinskey or Kuglen Hook can be inserted through the sideport incision to move the pupil away while doing capsulorhexis to achieve a larger sized rhexis.

- Sculpting is more difficult with small pupils as visualization is poor. The peripheral lens cannot be seen and the red reflex, which is required to visualize the depth of sculpting, is reduced by the smaller pupil diameter. These problems are overcome to a large extent using phaco chop techniques.
- For nucleus removal phaco chop, particularly vertical chop is the ideal technique in a miotic pupil, as it does not require a large pupil. Here, the phaco tip stays in the center of the pupil for the majority of the time, and the chances of capturing the iris or capsular edge is much lesser. The second instrument can be used to move the pupil away to get a perfect position and then phaco chop can be performed.
- An injector is preferred over the folding forceps for inserting the IOL. The tip of the folder may catch the iris in the presence of iris prolapse or a flaccid iris and cause a dialysis. The injector tip immediately plugs the incision and there will be a net influx of viscoelastic instead.
- An injector separates the IOL from the surrounding tissues keeping it sterile. It also helps in exact positioning of the IOL that is an advantage in a small pupil or a flaccid iris.
- As long as the tip of the injector fits into the capsulorhexis, the IOL can be delivered into the bag without stretching or tearing the capsulorhexis.
- The second instrument or viscoelastic can be used to push the iris back and away from the bevel of the injector where it might otherwise be caught.

- For the trailing haptic, two instruments can be used—one to hold the iris and the other to dial in the trailing haptic.
- With plate haptic IOLs, anterior capsular contracture is greater and there is also more giant cell reaction, hence older silicone IOLs should be avoided in eyes that are likely to be inflamed.
- Latest generation silicone IOLs such as Clariflex (AMO) has no difference in long-term inflammatory profiles between hydrophobic acrylic and second-generation silicone. The latest generation silicone achieved statistically significantly less inflammation than the AcrySof IOL in the long-term. The second- and higher-generation silicone IOLs are also more chemically pure and have a better overall design with a higher refractive index and thinner profile. Silicone IOLs also have a greater ease of implantation and reduced incision size as compared to acrylic IOLs.
- The unfolder Emerald injector allows the surgeon to use a full size 6-mm optic acrylic IOL in a three-piece model through a 3-mm incision.
- A Lister hook (Katena Products, Inc.) can be used in the second hand to retract the pupil to re-tear and enlarge a small capsulorhexis.
- Irrespective of the method chosen for enlarging the pupil during phacoemulsification, the pupil should be constricted at the end of surgery with an intraocular miotic. If necessary, the pupil should be stroked with a blunt, gentle instrument

to reduce its size. This prevents optic capture, capsular adhesion or other manner of pupillary deformity.
- Postoperatively, topical anti-inflammatory agents should be used to take care of the increased inflammatory activity secondary to increased maneuvering and longer and more difficult surgery.

SUBLUXATION OF THE LENS AND ITS MANAGEMENT

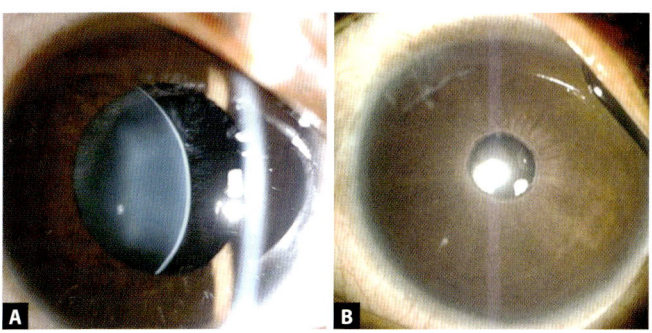

Figs 2.7A and B Subluxation of the lens. (A) Note the weakness of the zonular fibers and subluxation of the lens; (B) Postoperative photograph of the patient after glued IOL surgery

A: The surgical management of cataract associated with zonular dialysis (Fig. 2.7A) is a real challenge for the ophthalmic surgeon. Due to recent advances in equipment and instrumentation, better surgical techniques and understanding of the fluidics, the surgeon is able to perform relatively safe cataract surgery in presence of compromised zonules. Implantation of a capsular tension ring can stabilize a loose lens and allow the surgeon to complete phacoemulsification and IOL implantation.

The indication for use of capsular tension ring is in all cases of subluxation of lens ranging from the common ones like traumatic displacement (mechanical or surgical), Marfan's syndrome, pseudoexfoliation syndrome and hypermature cataract to the rare ones like aniridia and intraocular tumors. In severe cases, Cionni's ring is employed or even an endocapsular segment can be used.

B: The postoperative image of the same patient showing well centered IOL and round pupil (Fig. 2.7B).

MODIFIED CIONNI'S CAPSULAR TENSION RING

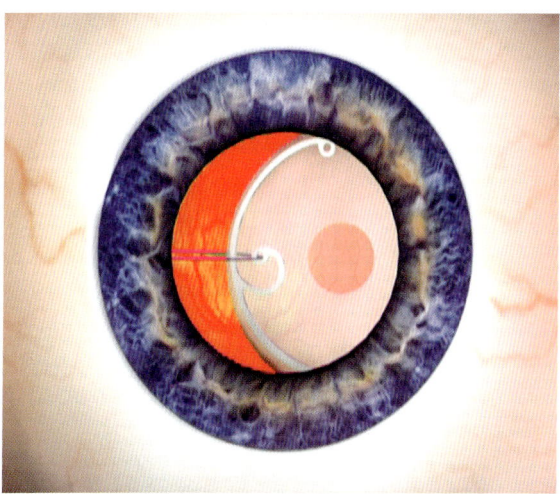

Fig. 2.8 Cionni's modified capsular tension ring being placed in position

Cionni's capsular tension ring (CTR) can be implanted in the eye after the completion of the capsulorhexis (Fig. 2.8). Some surgeons prefer putting it in the eye before phaco is begun whereas some surgeons prefer putting it after the phacoemulsification of the nucleus is completed.

Commencing capsulorhexis is difficult because of capsular instability. It is better to begin the capsulorhexis in the area where the zonules is whole and where the capsule offers sufficient resistance. If vitreous is present in the anterior chamber, the gel must be first isolated and vitrectomy should be performed if required. After the vitreous has been removed from the anterior chamber, a viscoelastic preferably dispersive is inserted by first covering the zone. Capsulorhexis can be performed after the zone of zonular dehiscence and iridocrystalline diaphragm have been stabilized. Do not use trypan blue in such cases as the trypan blue will go into the vitreous cavity through the zonular dehiscence and make the whole vitreous cavity blue. This will make visualization difficult in surgery. Completion of rhexis can be done using an intraocular rhexis forceps.

Cionni's CTR has an eyelet to which a 9-0 prolene suture is tied up and the CTR is fixed to the sclera with the help of suture. In cases of massive subluxation, even 2 Cionni's modified CTR can be placed in to the eye. Following this, a foldable IOL is injected in to the capsular bag as stability of the bag is now achieved.

LENTICULAR COLOBOMA

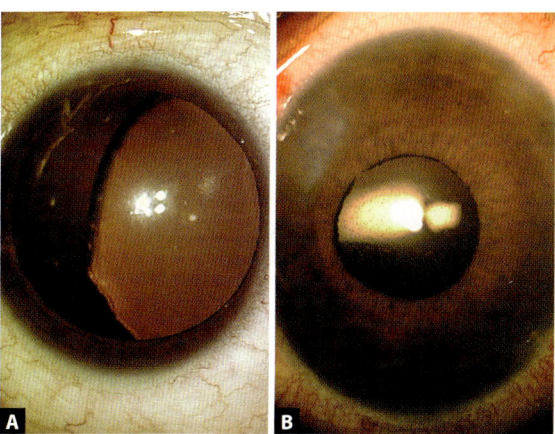

Figs 2.9A and B Massive lenticular coloboma. (A) Preoperative photograph; (B) Postoperative photograph after Glued IOL surgery was performed

A: Coloboma may occur as an isolated defect or as a feature of a variety of single-gene disorders, chromosomal syndromes, or malformation syndromes. Although not classically associated with Marfan's syndrome, colobomas have been described in several reports of Marfan's syndrome, typically involving the lens and rarely involving other ocular structures (Fig. 2.9A). A lens coloboma is not a true coloboma; it is just a zonular absence that causes a defect in the lens equator and hence a more spherical lens.

The underlying cause of the lens subluxation and zonular weakness in Marfan's syndrome is not eliminated by CTR implantation. Thus, further weakening of the zonules may occur in the long run, and, in the most unfortunate cases, may cause luxation of the capsular bag into the vitreous body. Lensectomy with vitrectomy is our preferred mode of handling such cases followed by secondary IOL fixation with Glued intrascleral fixation.

B: Postoperative image of the patient (Fig. 2.9B) following a Glued intrascleral haptic fixation of IOL (Glued IOL).

IRIS COLOBOMA

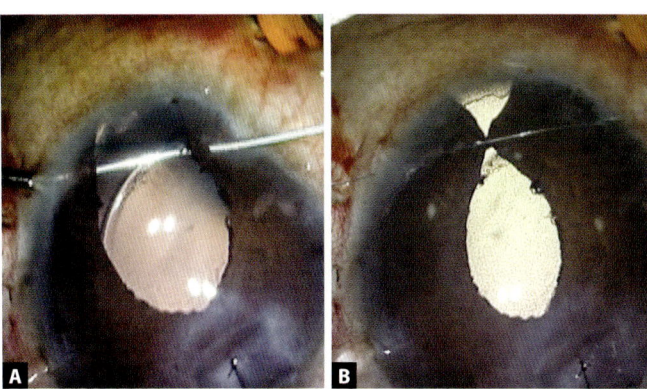

Figs 2.10A and B Iris coloboma. (A) Straight needle with 9-0 suture being passed. Modified Sieper's technique being performed; (B) Pupil reconstruction is done and suture is being tied

A: The image depicts a case of iris coloboma (Fig. 2.10A) where a Glued IOL surgery has been performed. Iris coloboma may exist as a separate entity or may be associated with a lens or choroidal coloboma.

The iris defect needs to be repaired to prevent visual disturbances to the patient. The most commonly employed method is to perform a modified Siepser's slip-knot technique to repair the iris defect.

B: Intraoperative image of the patient demonstrating the procedure of iris repair (Fig. 2.10B).

SOEMMERING RING

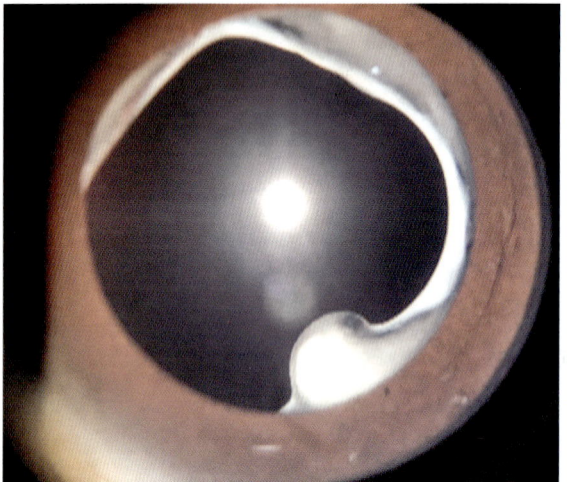

Fig. 2.11 Peripheral annular Soemmering ring

Soemmering ring (Fig. 2.11) is a type of 'after-cataract' that was first discovered by W Soemmering in the eyes of dead persons who underwent cataract surgery during their lifetime. It is the proliferation of lens material and cells in the eyes of pediatric patients who undergo cataract surgery.

Soemmering ring has a peripheral disposition and is often seen after the dilation of pupil. Although in some cases, it does get dislodged into the center of the pupil. In such cases it can be a cause of marked fall in visual acuity.

The treatment in these cases, calls for surgical removal of the Soemmering ring. If associated with a posterior capsule rupture, vitrectomy is done, care being taken not to dislodge the Soemmering ring. Following this a Glued IOL scaffold procedure is performed where in a 3-piece foldable IOL is injected beneath the Soemmering ring and the haptics are externalized as in a glued IOL procedure. The optic of the IOL acts as a scaffold and prevents the posterior dislodgement of the Soemmering ring. Phacoemulsification probe is introduced in to the eye and the Soemmering ring material is emulsified and removed from the eye.

In cases with intact posterior capsule, viscoexpression of the Soemmering ring material can be done from the eye followed by IOL implantation.

POSTERIOR LENTICONUS

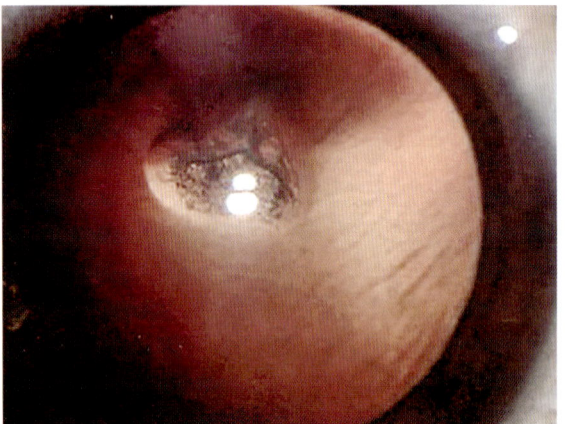

Fig. 2.12 Posterior lenticonus with associated cataract

Posterior lenticonus is a tricky situation that a surgeon faces and it can result in a devastation complication of dropped nucleus if not diagnosed and addressed properly. It is often associated with a typical 'Fish Tail' sign that is pathognomonic of an inherent defect present in the posterior capsule.

Posterior lenticonus is caused by thinning of the posterior capsule and gives a characteristic 'Oil droplet' appearance on red reflex examination (Fig. 2.12) . Precautions should be taken during the surgery. Hydrodissection should be avoided and phacoemulsification should be performed at low settings. The surgeon should be very carful during the irrigation-aspiration procedure due to thin posterior capsule. If a rupture occurs then posterior capsulorhexis should be attempted and vitrectomy should be done. The bag should be inflated with viscoelastic and a single piece IOL can be implanted in the bag or a 3-piece IOL can be implanted in the sulcus depending on the status of the capsular support present.

SECTION 3

Complications

Amar Agarwal
Priya Narang

SLEEVELESS PHACOTIP ASSISTED LEVITATION OF DROPPED NUCLEUS (SPAL) TECHNIQUE—STEP 1

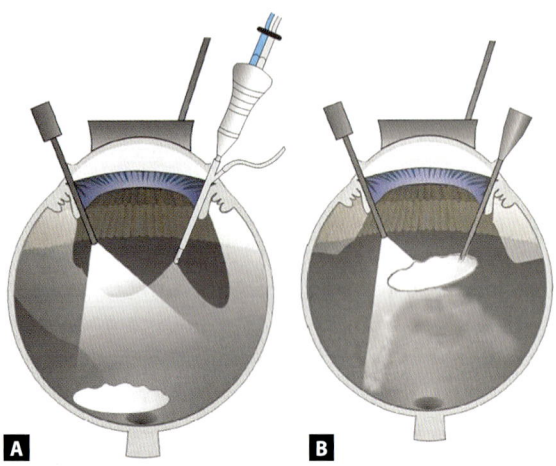

Figs 3.1A and B Sleeveless phacotip assisted levitation of dropped nucleus (SPAL). (A) The vitrectomy probe and endoilluminator are inserted through the standard 3 port pars plana incisions; (B) The vitrectomy probe is replaced by a sleeveless phaco probe (*Courtesy:* Clement Chan)

This innovative method was introduced by Agarwal et al. and was previously known as FAVIT. Its major advantage is that it allows the cataract surgeon familiar with vitreoretinal techniques to quickly convert over to posterior segment surgery with a limited amount of additional setup of instrumentation for removing the lens fragments. FAVIT stands for (FA—Fallen and VIT—Vitreous) meaning a technique to remove fragments fallen into the vitreous. A better term was then coined for this method and it came to be known as SPAL. Standard 3-port pars plana vitrectomy incisions are framed and an infusion cannula is fixated through the first port. An endoilluminator is then inserted through the second port (Fig. 3.1A), and a vitrectomy probe is inserted through the third port. Next, the surgeon performs a thorough posterior vitrectomy including the elimination of the vitreous fibers surrounding the retained lens fragments, in order to prevent subsequent vitreoretinal traction. After the completion of the posterior vitrectomy, the surgeon replaces the vitrectomy probe with a phacoemulsification probe (sleeveless) through the same incision. With the ultrasonic power at 50 percent and the aspiration intensity at moderate setting, the surgeon activates the suction-only mode to elevate the lens fragment from the retinal surface. A small burst of ultrasonic energy is applied to embed the probe tip into the elevated lens fragment, and then lifts the entire fragment anteriorly. The endoilluminator is also used at the same time to guide the lens fragment above the iris plane and into the anterior chamber (Fig. 3.1B). Once the lens fragment is in the anterior chamber, an IOL scaffold procedure can be performed where a 3-piece IOL is implanted below the lens fragments and is dialed over the residual capsular support. In cases of inadequate sulcus support, the IOL can even be placed above the iris and the nucleus can be emulsified. The optic of the IOL acts as scaffold and prevents any loss of lens fragments in to the posterior cavity. The same IOL can then be fixed in the eye by Glued IOL procedure. Stromal hydration is done to secure the corneal wound and air bubble is injected into the anterior chamber.

In cases of hard cataract, the corneal section can be enlarged and the nucleus can then be expelled from the eye as in a routine extracapsular cataract surgery.

A: After completing the anterior lenticular cortical clean up and anterior vitrectomy, posterior vitrectomy is performed. The vitrectomy probe and endoilluminator are inserted through separate clear corneal or scleral tunnel incisions created at the start of cataract surgery, and a vitrectomy contact lens is applied firmly on the cornea by surgical assistant to allow adequate viewing of the posterior fundus for the surgeon.

B: The vitrectomy probe is replaced with a phacoemulsification probe after completion of a posterior vitrectomy to engage the posteriorly dislocated nuclear lens fragment. Suction-only mode is activated to elevate the lens fragment, and the phaco tip is then embedded into the elevated lens fragment with a small burst of ultrasonic energy.

SPAL TECHNIQUE—STEP 2

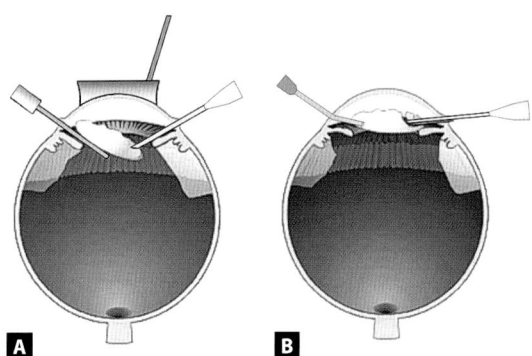

Figs 3.2A and B SPAL. (A) The dropped nuclear fragment is levitated into the anterior chamber; (B) The nuclear fragment is being emulsified in the anterior chamber
(*Courtesy*: Clement Chan)

A: The lens fragment is lifted anteriorly with the phaco probe while the endoilluminator is used at the same time to guide the lens fragment above the iris and into the anterior chamber (Fig. 3.2A).

B: Emulsification is performed on the lens fragment in the anterior chamber (Fig. 3.2B), while chopping and pulsing are avoided to prevent dropping smaller lens fragments back into the vitreous cavity.

DROPPED NUCLEUS LYING ON THE RETINA

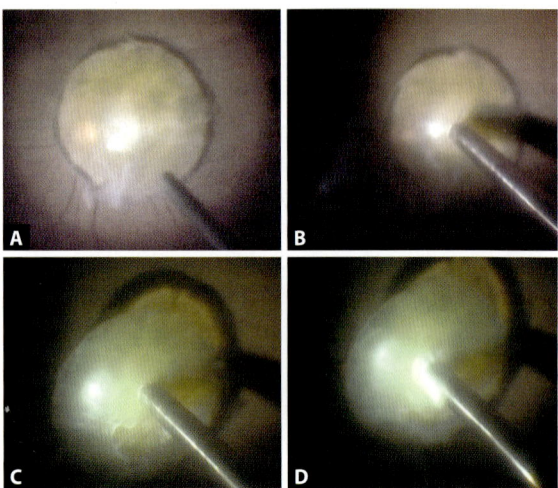

Figs 3.3A to D SPAL. (A) Thorough vitrectomy is done and the vitreous adhesions around the dropped nuclear fragments are released; (B) The sleeveless phaco probe is brought close to the dropped nucleus and vacuum is initiated; (C) The dropped fragment is lifted from the surface of retina; (D) When the fragment is lifted into the vitreous cavity the phaco probe is embedded into the nucleus by initiating the power mode. This prevents falling of the dropped fragment back on to the retina

The standard three-port pars plana vitrectomy approach is the most frequently employed method for the removal of posteriorly dislocated lens fragments in a safe and effective manner (Figs 3.3A to D). The first step involves the insertion of a posterior infusion cannula at the inferior temporal pars plana. In the event of a localized concomitant choroidal detachment in the inferior temporal quadrant, an alternative quadrant (e.g. inferior nasal) may be chosen for the infusion cannula. Frequently, cloudy media resulting from dense lens fragments or in some cases hyphema and fibrin deposits surrounding the implant, may prevent an adequate view of the tip of the pars plana infusion cannula. In that situation, the surgeon may ascertain the proper intravitreal location of the infusion cannula tip by inserting a micro-vitreoretinal blade through one of the superior pars plana sclerotomies to rub against the cannula tip, before turning on the infusion fluid. Utilizing a longer infusion cannula (e.g. 4- or 6 mm) is also advantageous in avoiding inadvertent subretinal or choroidal infusion.

MANAGING THE ANTERIOR CHAMBER OPACITIES AND HERNIATED VITREOUS

Cloudy lens material, hemorrhagic infiltrates, and fibrin deposits in the anterior chamber must be first eliminated before the performance of a posterior vitrectomy and phacofragmentation. For the anterior chamber washout, a separate infusion cannula (e.g. a 20- or 22-gauge angled rigid or flexible soft cannula) may be inserted at the limbus for anterior chamber infusion and prevention of chamber collapse. Microsurgical picks, hooks, bent needle tips, or forceps may be used to remove opaque membranes from the anterior and posterior surfaces of the implant. Vitreous herniated into the anterior chamber and vitreous strands attached to the iris or the limbal surgical wound must be excised with a vitrectomy probe in order to reduce the chance of postoperative cystoid macular edema and other types of vitreoretinal complications. To further enhance anterior media clarity, intracameral viscoelastic substances can be injected to coat the corneal endothelium for reducing striate keratopathy, displace blood from the visual axis, or to achieve hemostasis associated with a persistent hyphema. Unwanted residual lenticular capsular remnants may also be eliminated with the vitrectomy probe. Pupillary dilation may be maintained throughout surgery with the administration of topical and subconjunctival mydriatics, or intracameral epinephrine. If necessary, temporary iris retractors can be inserted via multiple limbal incisions to maintain pupillary dilation during surgery.

POSTERIOR VITRECTOMY AND PHACOFRAGMENTATION

After completing the core vitrectomy, it is important for the surgeon to carefully remove all of the vitreous fibers surrounding the posterior lens fragments before proceeding with phacofragmentation, in order to prevent the occlusion of the phaco tip by formed vitreous elements phacofragmentation process and also prevent traction on the retina. In fact, the surgeon should remove as much of the vitreous as he can safely achieve before performing phacoemulsification, in order to avoid unwanted vitreoretinal traction. Perfluorocarbon liquid may be infused into the eye to serve as a cushion for protecting the underlying retina from the bouncing lens fragments during the process of lens emulsification. Only a limited amount of perfluorocarbon liquid should be injected, since excessive perfluorocarbon liquid with a convex meniscus tends to displace the lens fragments away from the central visual axis and toward the peripheral fundus and the vitreous base. In case of peripheral displacement of the lens fragments, a layer of viscoelastic may be applied on top of the perfluorocarbon liquid to neutralize its convex meniscus, resulting in recentering of the lens fragments toward the visual axis, a simple maneuver described by Elizalde.

At the start of the pars plana phacoemulsification process, each lens fragment is first engaged at the phaco tip with the machine set at the aspiration mode and then brought to the mid vitreous cavity for emulsification. During the emulsification of the lens fragments, the ultrasonic power is kept at a low or moderate setting in order to decrease the tendency of blowing the fragments from the phaco tip and repeatedly dropping them on the retina. The more advanced phacofragmentation units with sophisticated linear (proportional) ultrasonic and aspiration controls tend to reduce the erratic movements of the lens fragments at the phaco tip during the fragmentation process. The surgeon may also stabilize a large lens fragment in the mid vitreous cavity by using his other hand to spear the fragment with an endoilluminator with a hook or pick at its tip for emulsification. As an alternative, he may utilize the bimanual "crush" or "chopstick" technique, which involves the use of his other hand to methodically crush each lens fragment with the tip of an endoilluminator against the phaco tip before aspirating it from the eye through the phaco tip. After emulsifying and removing the bulk of the lens fragments, the surgeon eliminates any remaining vitreous with the vitrectomy probe. He also carefully searches for and removes residual small lens fragments embedded at the vitreous base, as well as inspects the peripheral fundus with indirect ophthalmoscopy. One can use a combination of perflurocarbon liquids and FAVIT also. In this once vitrectomy is done PFCL is injected to raise the nuclear fragments from the retinal level. Then using the phaco needle they are removed. Retinal breaks and peripheral retinal detachment discovered during the inspection are then promptly treated with the appropriate modality (e.g. laser, cryotherapy, scleral buckling, fluid-air or gas exchange, etc.) Residual perfluorocarbon liquid is removed before closure. The postoperative therapy includes the application of topical steroidal or nonsteroidal anti-inflammatory medications, antibiotics, and cycloplegics.

INSULATING THE RETINA WITH PERFLUOROCARBON

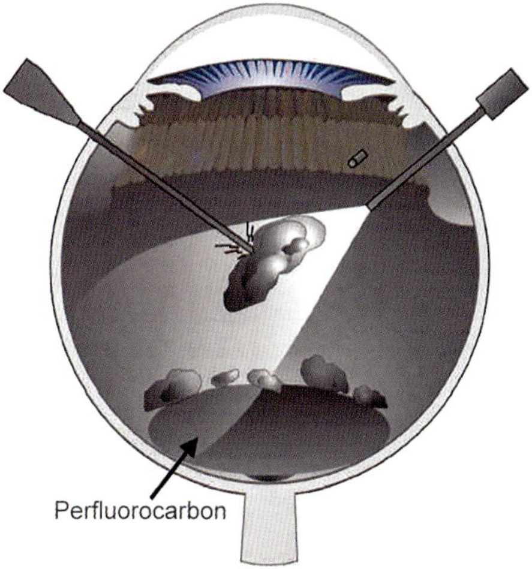

Fig. 3.4 Insulating the retina with perfluorocarbon (*Courtesy:* Clement Chan)

A small amount of perfluorocarbon liquid may be infused on the retinal surface to protect it from dropped lens fragments during the process of lens emulsification (Fig. 3.4). Excessive perfluorocarbon is avoided to decrease the propensity of peripheral displacement of the floating lens fragments toward the vitreous base due to the convex meniscus of the perfluorocarbon. During phacoemulsification, the ultrasonic power of the phaco probe is kept at a low to medium setting to reduce the tendency of blowing the lens fragments from the phaco tip toward the retina.

PRINCIPLE OF AN OPHTHALMIC ENDOSCOPIC SYSTEM

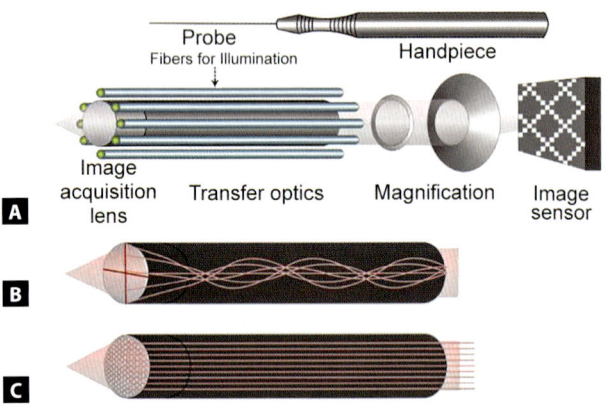

Figs 3.5A to C Principle of an ophthalmic endoscopic system
(*Courtesy:* Clement Chan)

The endoscopic approach is best suited for removing dislocated lens fragments from eyes with an opacified cornea, a miotic or occluded pupil, persistent hyphema, or a cloudy IOL, etc. It also provides a clear and unimpeded view of lens fragments trapped at the vitreous base. It allows the surgeon to scrutinize peripheral fundus details and appreciate the precise anatomical relationship of various retroirideal structures (e.g. iridocapsular interface, haptic-ciliary junction, vitreous base, etc.) The magnified and undistorted images of the peripheral intraocular structures provided by the endoscope cannot be obtained through other methods. The endoscopic system includes an endoscopic hand piece with a probe, connected to a fiberoptic light source, a charged coupled device (CCD) video camera system and recorder, coupled with a high-resolution color video monitor. For optimal viewing, a bright light source such as Xenon is preferred, although halogen lights can be used. The two types of ophthalmic endoscopic systems that are commercially available include the gradient Index (GRIN) solid-rod endoscopes first developed by Eguchi, and the fiberoptic endoscopes subsequently developed by Uram and Fisher. Both types of devices share the principle of image acquisition and optics transfer through the distal probe, and then image magnification and coupling in the handpiece or the remote CCD camera unit (Fig. 3.5A). The GRIN solid rod endoscope employs a single long, slender, glass lens for optics transfer. The image acquired at the probe is transmitted along the length of a cylindrical pathway of the solid lens with a gradient index in a sinusoidal mode to a CCD camera unit (Fig. 3.5B). The index of refraction of the lens varies with the distance from the central axis. In the case of a fiberoptic endoscope, the image acquired with a GRIN lens at the distal end of a handpiece is transferred through a bundle of microfibers (via total internal reflection within each fiber) to a CCD camera unit (Fig. 3.5C). The fiberoptic endoscope allows for a lighter handpiece. However, its image resolution is limited by the pixel density of the CCD camera as well as the density of the microfibers, and its depth of field is less than the GRIN single-rod endoscope. Besides vitrectomy and phacoemulsification, other surgical maneuvers including laser photocoagulation can be performed in conjunction with the endoscopic system. Laser componentry can be built into the endoscopic system. For instance, the endoscopic hand piece may contain an optical path for viewing, besides separate fibers for endoillumination and photocoagulation. Thus a single endoscopic handpiece can be constructed with the capability of performing multiple tasks simultaneously: viewing, endoillumination, and photocoagulation. Even a channel for infusion can also be incorporated into the endoscope. However, the multiple functions increase the bulk and weight of the hand piece. One commercially available fiberoptic endoscopic system offers a 20-gauge endoscopic hand piece with a 3000-pixel fiberoptic bundle allowing a 70-degree field of view and a depth of focus from 0.5 to 7.0 mm, or an18-gauge hand piece with a 10,000-pixel fiberoptic bundle allowing a 110-degree field of view and a depth of focus from 1 to 20 mm. Drawbacks of the endoscopic method include the lack of a stereoscopic or three-dimensional view, and an initially steep learning curve for the surgeon. Excellent surgical results can be achieved with this technique. In their study published in 1998, Boscher and associates reported consistently successful outcome in the use of the endoscopic method for managing a consecutive series of 30 eyes with dislocated lens fragments or IOLs.

Further development in ophthalmic endoscopic systems holds the promise of providing unparalleled microscopic images of intraocular structures (even on a cellular level) that are not possible through conventional surgical instrumentation (e.g. viewing of sensory retinal, retinal pigment epithelial, and choroidal components in the subretinal space during vitreoretinal surgery). The construction of stereoscopic endoscopes is also technically feasible.

REMOVAL OF ENTIRE HARD LENS FRAGMENT WITH PERFLUOROCARBON

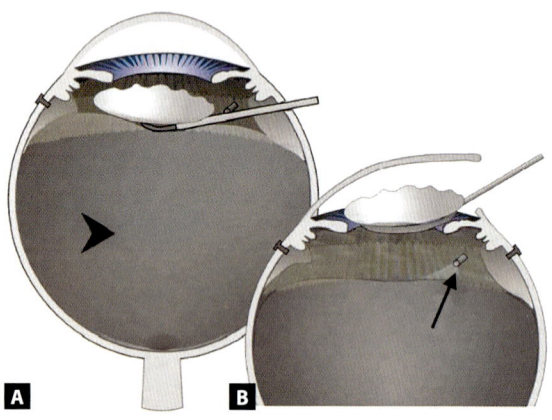

Figs 3.6A and B Removal of entire hard lens fragment with perfluorocarbon
(Courtesy: *Clement Chan*)

High density, inert behavior, and low viscosity are unique properties of perfluorocarbon liquid that allow its use as an elegant surgical tool for removing dislocated lens fragments with minimal instrumentation in a safe and consistent manner. As described in the previous section, perfluorocarbon liquid is frequently used to insulate the retina from injury by dropped lens fragments during phacoemulsification. Perfluorocarbon is particularly effective when the surgeon is faced with the adverse condition of poor visibility through a hazy cornea and a dislocated nucleus with a rock-hard consistency. In that situation, he may use perfluorocarbon alone without phacoemulsification to deliver the lens fragment anteriorly for its extraction through a limbal wound. Employing conventional phacoemulsification techniques to retrieve a hard lens nucleus may be time consuming and hazardous, particularly in the presence of marked ocular inflammation and a cloudy media with poor visibility. Historically, several methods of removing a dislocated hard nucleus were utilized in the past. With the exception of cryoextraction, these methods have been largely abandoned due to their technical difficulties and associated potential complications. They include trapping the lens nucleus with two needles passed across the globe with the patient in a prone position and buoying the lens nucleus anteriorly with sodium hyaluronate. The needle-trapping technique is inherently difficult to apply and is associated with many potential hazards. Although sodium hyaluronate is well tolerated by the eye, its relatively low density in comparison to perfluorocarbon does not allow the buoying of the lens nucleus on a consistent basis. In contrast to perfluorocarbon liquid, clear visibility is required for the precise placement of the sodium hyaluronate with a cannula under the dislocated nucleus in order for it to float the nucleus. To avoid the premature dilution and extrusion of the sodium hyaluronate from the globe, the infusion fluid must also be turned off temporarily during the placement of the sodium hyaluronate. Such a maneuver may lead to hypotony and miosis with potentially serious consequences during surgery. For the above reasons, perfluorocarbon liquid is superior to sodium hyaluronate and is currently the agent of choice for floating a posteriorly dislocated lens fragment for removal.

Shapiro and associates reported the removal of dislocated hard lens nuclei with perfluoro-n-octane in 1991 (Figs 3.6A and B). Their technique includes an initial vitrectomy to eliminate vitreoretinal traction after a thorough clean up of the anterior lenticular cortical and capsular remnants. The subsequent intraocular infusion of perfluoro-n-octane floats the hard lens nucleus anteriorly toward the vitreous base. The nuclear fragment is displaced peripherally due to the convex meniscus of the perfluorocarbon, and temporarily wedged at the vitreous base between the surface of the perfluorocarbon and the iris and ciliary processes. No attempt is made to directly expulse the dislocated lens fragment into the anterior chamber and out of the limbal wound with the perfluorocarbon liquid, due to potential mechanical injury of the corneal endothelium and the iris by the hard lens nucleus with such a maneuver. Instead, a soft-tipped cannula is inserted through a sclerotomy to recenter the lens nucleus behind the pupil (Fig. 3.6A). The lens nucleus is then gently floated further anteriorly with slow infusion of balanced salt solution on top of the perfluorocarbon, and carefully brought into the anterior chamber for delivery out of the eye with a lens loop through a limbal incision

(Fig. 3.6B). In the absence of poor integrity of the cornea and the iris, a secondary IOL can be conveniently implanted through the same limbal incision before closure. Due to its low viscosity and tendency for posterior pooling, the surgeon can easily remove the perfluorocarbon liquid with a small aspiration cannula after the closure of the limbal wound at the end of surgery. Besides Shapiro's report, there have been a series of reports by multiple surgeons in the effective use of a variety of perfluorocarbon liquids to remove dislocated intraocular lens fragments. Similar to cryoextraction, this method of removing lens fragments is not appropriate for an eye with an IOL, unless the IOL is explanted first or at the time of the lens fragment removal.

The special properties of perfluorocarbon liquid make it especially suitable as an intraocular tool for atraumatic tissue manipulation when the surgeon encounters the situation of posteriorly dislocated lens fragments in conjunction with retinal breaks and a retinal detachment. In the presence of a giant retinal tear or a large retinal dialysis, perfluorocarbon frequently becomes indispensable for a successful surgical outcome. The retinal complications may be related to pre-existing retinal pathology, elicited by vitreoretinal traction associated with attempts to remove the lens fragments during the primary cataract surgery, or retinal injury from the dropped lens fragments subsequently. The retinal breaks may also enlarge and a retinal detachment may progress during the process of lens fragment removal. In such a situation, perfluorocarbon liquid serves the dual purpose of stabilizing the retinal complications and preventing more retinal injury, while the lens fragments are floated anteriorly for phacoemulsification or removal through a limbal incision. Any posterior hemorrhage from the retinal breaks may also be displaced anteriorly by the perfluorocarbon liquid for removal. With the retina held down by the perfluorocarbon liquid, standard vitreoretinal techniques are employed to repair the retinal breaks and detachment following the vitrectomy and elimination of the lens fragments. After the application of laser or cryotherapy and possible placement of a scleral buckle, fluid-air or gas exchange is performed to replace the perfluorocarbon liquid and to achieve appropriate retinal tamponade. In case of proliferative vitreoretinopathy, silicone oil may be required as the agent for prolonged retinal tamponade. Utilizing perfluorocarbon liquid in a manner similar to the above description, Lewis and others reported favorable outcome in managing dislocated lens fragments and IOLs. Improved care and methods in the management of dislocated lens fragments during the primary cataract extraction and the subsequent surgery may be responsible for the much lower prevalence of associated retinal breaks and detachment in recent reports in contrast to earlier studies (3% to 5% versus 7% to 50%.) In a recent study, Moore and colleagues reported a combined incidence of 13.4% for retinal detachment associated with retained lens fragments and their subsequent surgical management (6.4% before pars plana vitrectomy and 7.0% after pars plana vitrectomy).

MANAGEMENT OF LENS COLOBOMA WITH GLUED IOL

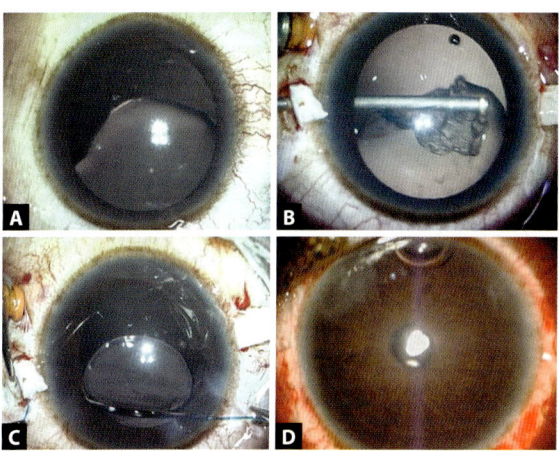

Figs 3.7A to D Management of massive lens coloboma. (A) Lenticular coloboma; (B) Two partial scleral thickness scleral flaps made as in a glued IOL surgery. Lensectomy with vitrectomy being performed; (C) 3-piece foldable IOL is injected and the leading haptic is externalized as in a glued IOL surgery; (D) Postoperative image of the eye on third postop day. Note the presence of an air bubble in the anterior chamber

The term 'Coloboma' is derived from the Greek word 'Koloboma' which means a 'hole'. Coloboma of lens (Fig. 3.7A) is usually unilateral but in some cases bilateral and double coloboma may be present. The zonules may be maldeveloped, which may be due to either typically incomplete closure of the optic vesicle, or it may be due to persistent remnants of fibro vascular sheath of the lens interfering with development of zonules.

Coloboma may occur as an isolated defect or as a feature of a variety of single-gene disorders, chromosomal syndromes, or malformation syndromes. Although not classically associated with Marfan syndrome, colobomas have been described in several reports of Marfan syndrome, typically involving the lens and rarely involving other ocular structures. A lens coloboma is not a true coloboma; it is just a zonular absence that causes a defect in the lens equator and hence a more spherical lens.

These cases require adequate preoperative workup in the form of posterior segment examination and calculation of the corrective IOL power as these cases may be associated with colobomas of the macula and optic disc. The IOL power calculation in such cases is often guided by the patient's refraction and by measuring the distance to the patients preferred fixation. The patients often present with poor vision resulting from peripheral lenticular astigmatism and glare.

These are potentially surgically challenging cases, which often necessitate the use of capsular tension rings (CTR) and endocapsular segments (ECS). Other problem associated with such cases is the intraoperative challenge of fixing the CTR and ECS along with prevention of the vitreous herniation in to the anterior chamber. The postoperative challenges of IOL decentration and capsular phimosis and degradation of suture also defy the success of performing a surgery. To overcome all these sticky situations, a glued IOL surgery is performed but that too has its own set of limitations especially in big eyes as in a case of marfans syndrome.

The surgery proceeds with the making of two partial scleral thickness scleral flaps and performing lensectomy with vitrectomy (Fig. 3.7B) as in a normal glued IOL surgery. Following the externalization of haptics (Fig. 3.7C), scleral pockets are created with a 26 G needle parallel to the sclerotomy incision along the edge of the bed of flap. Haptics are tucked in to these pockets and vitrectomy is performed at the sclerotomy site. Fibrin glue is applied beneath the flaps and the conjunctiva to seal all the openings. The postoperative results of glued IOL (Fig. 3.7D) are very encouraging in these cases.

DISLOCATED IOL ON THE RETINA

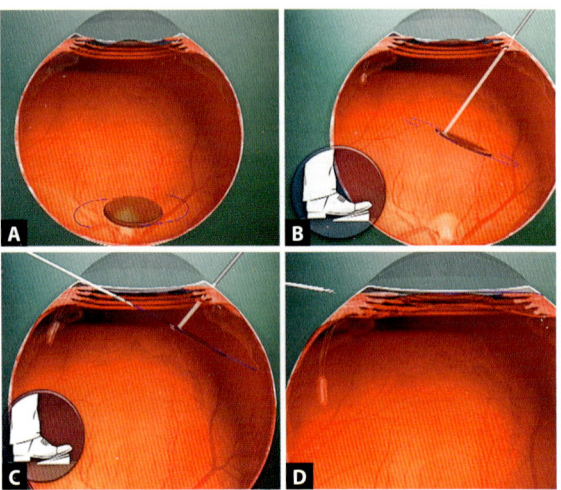

Figs 3.8A to D Sleeveless extrusion cannula assisted levitation of dropped IOL. (A) Image shows a dropped IOL lying on the retinal surface; (B) After thorough vitrectomy, vacuum is initiated and the IOl is lifted with a sleeveless extrusion cannula; (C) IOL is levitated and is brought in to the mid pupillary plane; (D) The IOL is then explanted or repositioned in to the eye depending on the presence or absence of sulcus support and also upon the type of IOL levitated

SLEEVELESS EXTRUSION CANNULA FOR LEVITATION OF DROPPED IOL

Dislocation of an intraocular lens in to the posterior chamber is a dreaded complication of modern cataract surgery as there is a continuous tussle to optimize the visual outcome and meet the expectations of a highly demanding patient. Since first described by Flynn et al. the soft-tipped extrusion cannula has been commonly used to drain the posterior subretinal fluid. The flexible silicone tubing attached to the end of a tapered extrusion needle is advanced into the subretinal space through an open peripheral break to allow drainage of posterior subretinal fluid atraumatically. These cannulas facilitate atraumatic drainage of subretinal fluid through pre-existing retinal holes and tears or through a retinotomy performed during vitreoretinal microsurgery. Addressing the IOL with extrusion cannula without sleeves gives a larger surface area to be adhered to the IOL and when this is followed by application of adequate suction, an IOL can be lifted and brought in to the pupillary plane from where it can be grasped by a forceps and then subsequently removed.

SURGICAL TECHNIQUE

Under local anesthesia, standard 23 gauge 3-port pars plana vitrectomy incisions are framed and the initial step is complete removal of the vitreous by thorough vitrectomy to prevent traction on the retina from subsequent maneuvers. After release of all the vitreo-lenticular adhesions, complete vitrectomy with careful separation and removal of the posterior hyaloid face is performed prior to lifting the IOL. The IOL gently floats to the posterior pole of the eye, once it is freed from all attachments (Fig. 3.8A).

The sleeveless-extrusion cannula is then connected to the vitreotome and the vacuum is set to 300 mm Hg, with the cutting function turned off. As the IOL rests flat on the retina, the sleeveless extrusion cannula is made to face the center of the optic and suction is initiated. The suction can be dynamically controlled with the foot pedal. The linear control of the foot pedal helps to increase the vacuum as and when needed during the levitation of IOL (Fig. 3.8B). Ineffective apposition of the lumen of the cannula to the surface of the IOL optic can lead to loss of vacuum. The IOL is lifted from the surface of the retina and is brought into the anterior vitreous in the mid-pupillary area (Fig. 3.8C). The end-opening forceps introduced from the corneal incision under direct visualization through the microscope grasps the IOL; the extrusion cannula is then removed as the forceps grasps the IOL. The IOL can then be subsequently managed depending on the surgical scenario. It can be either replaced or re-positioned in the sulcus or it can be explanted (Fig. 3.8D).

Various methods have been described in the peer review literature for levitation of dropped intraocular lenses. Retinal forceps is often used and is usually the standard mainstay of treatment in vitreoretinal surgery. Accidental creation of an iatrogenic retinal tear while lifting an IOL from the surface of the retina is always a possibility with its use. Often the IOLs are sneaky, slippery and difficult to grasp especially in cases of plate haptic IOLs.

The flexible silicon sleeve fits snugly within the rigid outer shaft of the cannula to prevent an air or fluid leakage around the outside of the cannula and provides better access due to its flexibility into the subretinal space. Removal of the silicon sleeve exposes wider access of the bore of the cannula, which helps to create an effective suction around the IOL.

The advantage with this technique is that it is safe, reliable and reproducible. Moreover, it is effective for dislocation of any type of IOL including the plate haptic IOLs which are often difficult to grasp with a retinal forceps. Another advantage is that no additional device is required and inaccessibility or unavailability of the device is not an issue as it is virtually present in all the vitreoretinal surgeons setup.

Numerous advances in microsurgical techniques have led to highly safe and effective cataract surgery. Two of the current trends in the evolution of modern cataract techniques include increasingly smaller surgical incisions associated with phacoemulsification (e.g. sub 1.4 mm incisions as in Phakonit with rollable IOL implantation), as well as the movement from retrobulbar and peribulbar anesthesia to topical anesthesia, and even "no anesthesia" techniques. Despite such advances, the malpositioning or dislocation of an intraocular lens (IOL) due to capsular rupture or zonular dehiscence remains an infrequent but important sight-threatening complication for contemporary cataract surgery. The key to the prevention of poor visual outcome for this complication is its proper management.

Many highly effective surgical methods have been developed to manage a dislocated IOL. They include manipulating the IOL with perfluorocarbon liquids, scleral loop fixation, using a snare, employing 25-gauge IOL forceps, temporary haptic externalization, as well as managing the one-piece plate IOL and two simultaneous intraocular implants.

PERFLUOROCARBON LIQUIDS

Chang popularized the use of perfluorocarbon liquids for the surgical treatment of various vitreoretinal disorders. Due to their heavier-than-water properties, and their ease of intraocular injection and removal, perfluorocarbon liquids are highly effective for flattening detached retina, tamponading retinal tears, limiting intraocular hemorrhage, as well as floating dropped crystalline lens fragments and a dislocated IOL.

Types of Perfluorocarbon Liquids

Four types of perfluorocarbon liquids are frequently employed for intraocular surgery. They include:
1. Perfluoro-N-Octane
2. Perfluoro-Tributylamine
3. Perfluoro-Decaline
4. Perfluoro-Phenanthrene
   Their physical properties are outlined in Table 3.1.

Table 3.1 Properties of perfluorocarbon liquids				
Characteristic	Perfluoro-n Octane	Perfluoro-Tributylamine	Perfluoro-Decaline	Perfluoro-phenanthrene
Chemical formula	C3F18	C12F27N	C10F18	C14F24
Molecular weight	438	671	462	624
Specific gravity	1.76	1.89	1.94	2.03
Refractive index	1.27	1.29	1.31	1.33
Surface tension (Dyne/cm at 25°C)	14	16	16	16
Viscosity (Centistokes—25°C)	0.8	2.6	2.7	8.03
Vapor pressure (mm Hg at 37°C)	50	1.14	13.5	<1

IOL Manipulation with Perfluorocarbon Liquids

Due to their unique physical properties, perfluorocarbon liquids are well suited for floating dropped lens fragments and dislocated IOL, in order to insulate the underlying retina from damages. At the same time, the anterior displacement of the dislocated IOL by the perfluorocarbon liquids facilitates its removal or repositioning.

25-G CHANG PASSIVE-ACTION IOL FORCEPS

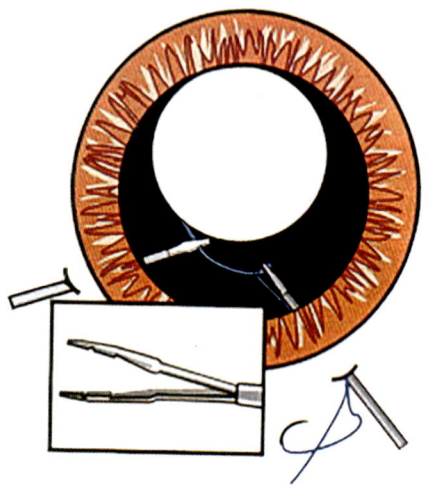

Fig. 3.9 25-G Chang passive-action IOL forceps
(*Courtesy:* Clement Chan)

In 1994, Chang introduced the 25-gauge IOL forceps. His passive-action forceps have smooth platforms at the distal end for grasping tissue or holding a suture, and a small groove at the proximal end for gripping a haptic. After a partial vitrectomy, a sharp 25-gauge, 5/8 inch needle is inserted through a scleral groove at 0.8 mm posterior to the corneoscleral limbus, to create a tract for the 25-gauge forceps. The forceps holding a slip-knot (lasso) on a 10-0 polypropylene suture is then inserted through the grooved scleral incision into the eye for engaging an IOL haptic. After looping the haptic, the forceps are released from the suture and are used to regrasp the end of the haptic; thus preventing the suture from slipping off the haptic. After tightening the slip knot, the IOL is repositioned in the ciliary sulcus by anchoring the needle of the 10-0 polypropylene suture within the scleral groove (Fig. 3.9). The same maneuver may be repeated for the opposite haptic, if necessary. The scleral groove is closed with an interrupted 10-0 nylon suture.

TEMPORARY HAPTIC EXTERNALIZATION

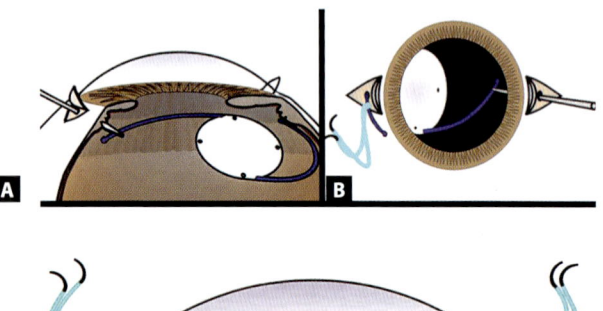

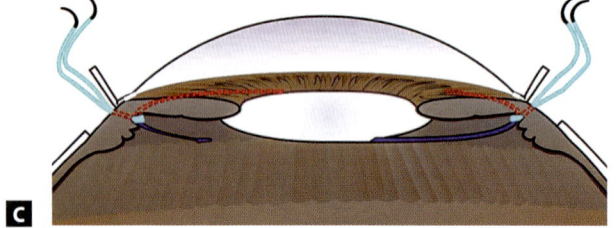

Figs 3.10A to C Temporary haptic externalization
(*Courtesy:* Clement Chan)

Chan first described this method in 1992. Its main features involve temporary haptic externalization for suture placement after a pars plana vitrectomy, followed by reinternalization of the haptics tied with 9-0 or 10-0 polypropylene sutures for secured anchoring by the anterior sclerotomies. The details of this technique include the following:
- A 3-port pars plana vitrectomy is performed for the removal of the anterior and central vitreous adjacent to the dislocated

IOL, in order to prevent any vitreoretinal traction during the process of manipulating the IOL.
- Two diametrically opposed limbal-based partial thickness triangular scleral flaps are prepared along the horizontal meridians at 3 and 9 o'clock. Anterior sclerotomies within the beds under the scleral flaps are made at 1 to 1.5 mm from the limbus (Fig. 3.10A). As an alternative to the scleral flaps, the anterior sclerotomies may be made within scleral grooves at 1 to 1.5 mm from the horizontal limbus.
- A fiberoptic light pipe is inserted through one of the posterior sclerotomies, while a pair of fine non-angled positive action forceps (e.g. Grieshaber 612.8) is inserted through the anterior sclerotomy of the opposing quadrant to engage one haptic of the dislocated IOL for temporary externalization (Fig. 3.10B). A double-armed 9-0 (Ethicon TG 160-8 plus, Somerville NJ) or 10-0 polypropylene suture (Ethicon CS 160-6 Somerville NJ) is tied around the externalized haptic to make a secured knot. The same process is repeated for the other haptic after the surgeon switches the instruments to his opposite hands.
- The externalized haptics with the tied sutures are re-internalized through the corresponding anterior sclerotomies with the same forceps (Fig. 3.10C). The surgeon anchors the internalized haptics securely in the ciliary sulcus by taking scleral bites with the external suture needles on the lips of the anterior sclerotomies. By adjusting the tension of

the opposing sutures while tying the polypropylene suture knots by the anterior sclerotomies, the optic is centered behind the pupil, and the haptics are anchored in the ciliary sulcus.

Several important features of this technique include:

- The horizontal meridians are chosen for the location of the anterior sclerotomies for easier manipulation of the forceps, haptics and sutures during the repositioning process.
- The locations of the anterior sclerotomies determine the final position of the IOL. Previous anatomic studies have reported the ciliary sulcus to be between 0.46 mm to 0.8 mm from the limbus. Thus the distance of 1 mm to 1.5 mm from the limbus places the anterior sclerotomies close to the external surface of the ciliary sulcus. Making the anterior sclerotomies at less than 1 mm from the limbus increases the risk of injuring the anterior chamber angle or the iris root.
- The following steps are taken to ease the passage of the Haptics through the anterior sclerotomies and reduce the chance of haptic breakage: (a) The anterior sclerotomies should have adequate size. If necessary, they may be widened before haptic reinternalization. (b) Fine non-angled positive action intraocular forceps are used for the haptic manipulation to give the surgeon the maximal "feel" and "control". Excessive pinching of the haptics is avoided during the passage of the haptics.

Several measures may also be taken to prevent the decentering and tilting of the IOL:
- The anterior sclerotomies are made at 180° from each other.
- The sutures are tied at equal distance from the ends of both haptics.
- *A four-point-fixation option*: To enhance more stability, two separate polypropylene sutures can be tied on each haptic, and the associated needles are anchored on the two "corners" of each anterior sclerotomy. This allows a stable configuration of four-point fixation of the IOL.

This repositioning technique combines the best features of the external and the internal approaches, while avoiding any intricate and cumbersome intraocular manipulations. With the easy placement of the anchoring sutures in an "opened" environment and the maintenance of the integrity of the globe in a "closed" environment, this technique allows a precise and secured fixation of the dislocated IOL in the ciliary sulcus on a consistent basis.

REMOVAL OF A PLATE HAPTIC IOL

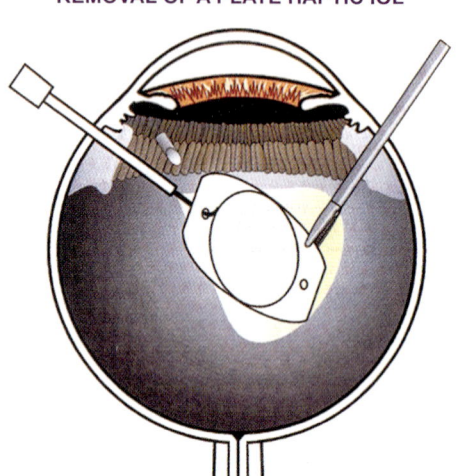

Fig. 3.11 Removal of a plate haptic IOL
(*Courtesy:* Clement Chan)

The slippery plate implant may be lifted on its edge or hooked through a positioning hole with a lighted pick, and then grasped with intraocular forceps for its repositioning or removal.

There is a lack of fibrous adhesion between the lens capsule and the one-piece silicone IOL with plate haptics even years after its insertion into the capsular bag. The "slippery" surface of the one-piece silicone plate implant makes it relatively mobile, even years after its placement. The silicone plate implant is fixated in the capsular bag by capsular contraction. After its implantation, there is fibrotic fusion of the anterior and posterior capsules as well as capsular purse-stringing due to anterior capsular contraction. These effects induce the posterior bowing of the silicone plate implant against the posterior capsule, resulting in the posterior capsular tightening and stretching. Thus any dehiscence of the capsular bag outside of the capsulorhexis allows the release of the "built-up" tension, and the expulsion of the implant through the dehiscence. Frequently, further capsular contraction after a posterior YAG capsulotomy may then vault the one-piece silicone plate implant through the opening into the vitreous cavity, in a delayed fashion.

Previous reports have advocated the repositioning of the dislocated silicone plate implant anterior to the capsular remnants or in the ciliary sulcus. Schneiderman and Johnson described the technique of picking the slippery silicone plate implant off the retinal surface with a lighted pick. The surgeon extends the tip of the pick under the edge of the silicone plate implant to gently elevate it off the retinal surface. The elevated edge is then grasped with the intraocular forceps for the repositioning or removal of the implant. Alternatively, the plate implant may be brought anteriorly by hooking the lighted pick through one of its positioning holes, and then grasped with forceps at the anterior or mid-vitreous cavity (Fig. 3.11). Another method is to aspirate the plate implant with a soft-tip cannula. As discussed above, perfluorocarbon liquids may also be used to float the dislocated plate implant. The one-piece silicone plate implant is designed for insertion into the capsular bag. Thus repositioning the silicone plate implant anterior to the capsular remnants or in the ciliary sulcus tends to be unstable, particularly without the support of sutures. None of the suturing methods (including the temporary haptic externalization technique described) work well for the one-piece silicone IOL with plate haptics. The temporary externalization of the bulky plate haptics of the silicone plate implant is awkward, and the suture placement through its "floppy" surface tends to result in the "cheese-wiring" of the implant. Frequently, the best approach for managing the dislocated one-piece silicone plate implant is its removal.

MANAGEMENT OF EYES WITH TWO INTRAOCULAR IMPLANTS

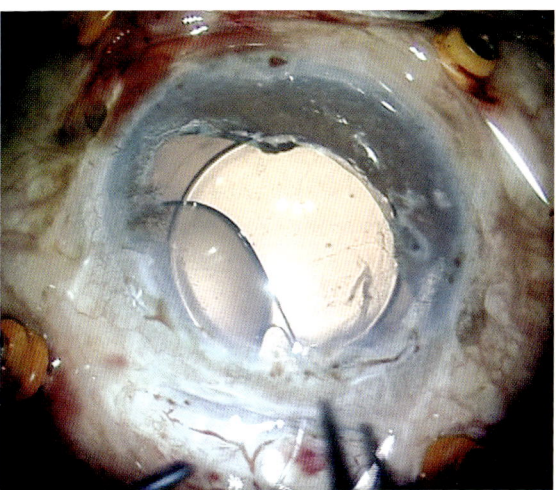

Fig. 3.12 Management of eyes with two intraocular implants. Note a well-placed IOL along with a second IOL being explanted from the edges of the previously placed IOL through a scleral tunnel

The presence of two intraocular implants complicates the surgical management. This usually occurs when the cataract surgeon inserts a second implant (usually an AC IOL) without removing the posteriorly dislocated implant. If a dislocated implant is made out of relatively soft and inert material (e.g. one-piece silicone implant with plate haptics), it may not cause a retinal injury. In that situation, surgical intervention may be avoided, although intraocular movements of the loose implant may create a visual disturbance. Mobile dislocated implants with hard surfaces and sharp edges may induce an intraocular injury, and therefore should be removed. The association of vitreous hemorrhage, glaucoma, uveitis, retinal breaks, or a retinal detachment with the dislocated implant also requires surgical intervention. The presence of the second intraocular implant eliminates the option of repositioning the dislocated implant, and it also interferes with the removal of the dislocated implant. A number of techniques have been described in the removal of the dislocated implant in the presence of a second implant. The dislocated implant may be treated as an intraocular foreign body, and removed through a pars plana incision with standard vitreoretinal techniques, as reported by Williams et al. The dislocated implant may also be removed through a limbal incision with or without the simultaneous removal of the second implant. Wong recently described a technique of temporarily suspending the dislocated implant at the anterior vitreous cavity by passing a 6-0 nylon suture through one of the IOL positioning holes; followed by gently tilting up the edge of the second implant to allow the delivery of the dislocated implant out of the eye through a limbal incision. Another option is the removal of the second implant followed by the repositioning of the dislocated implant. This option may be chosen if there is marked anterior segment pathology associated with a second anterior chamber implant (marked iridodialysis or hyphema, progressive corneal edema, etc.), and the dislocated posterior chamber implant can be safely fixated in the ciliary sulcus. Another option is the removal of both implants, particularly when the presence of any implant may aggravate a serious ocular condition; such as poorly controlled glaucoma, or an advanced retinal detachment with severe proliferative vitreoretinopathy. Whether the removal of one or both implants is through a limbal or pars plana opening, a relatively large incision is required, and complex maneuvers are necessary. This increases the chance of ocular morbidities. Thus the placement of a second implant should be avoided in the setting of a posteriorly dislocated implant.

In the Figure 3.12, the patient underwent a glued IOL fixation of an IOL and it was later discovered that a previous IOL was present in the subscleral space and it was missed in the preoperative examination. In this case, the IOL was dislodged from the subscleral space and delivered in to the posterior segment. The IOL was then manipulated carefully around the edges of the glued IOL and delivered in to the anterior chamber from where it was explanted.

ENDOPHTHALMITIS: METHODS OF COLLECTING SPECIMENS

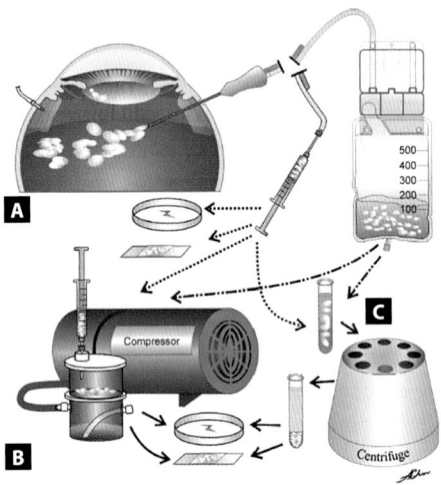

Figs 3.13A to C Endophthalmitis: Methods of collecting specimens
(*Courtesy:* Clement Chan)

- **A:** Undiluted aqueous and vitreous specimens may be directly inoculated onto culture media and used for smear preparation
- **B:** Diluted vitreous specimen collected into a syringe or a cassette is either first concentrated by vacuuming the diluted fluid in a sterile upper chamber through a 0.45-μm membrane filter into a lower sterile chamber **(suction filter method)**

C: Concentrated in a sterile centrifuge tube after performing high-speed centrifuge **(centrifuge method)**. Small cut segments of the membrane filter with the concentrated specimens or the sediments from the centrifuged tube are inoculated into culture media and applied on slides for smear preparation.

Despite numerous recent advances in its treatment, infectious endophthalmitis continues to be one of the most serious complications in ophthalmology. The infectious organism associated with endophthalmitis causes prominent ocular inflammation and toxic reaction, leading to severe intraocular tissue damages and the consequential marked visual loss. Infectious endophthalmitis can be broadly divided into five types: (1) Acute or early-onset postoperative (usually after cataract extraction), (2) Chronic or late-onset, (3) Bleb-related, (4) Post-traumatic, and (5) Endogenous or metastatic. The majority of endophthalmitis cases encountered by the practicing clinician consist of the first type: acute endophthalmitis after cataract extraction and intraocular lens (IOL) insertion However, any ocular surgery, including the relatively "non-penetrating" ones (e.g. strabismus, refractive procedures, trans-scleral fixation of a posterior chamber implant-PCIOL) may result in endophthalmitis.

CLINICAL FEATURES

The preliminary diagnosis of acute postoperative bacterial endophthalmitis must be based on clinical grounds alone, so that the clinician may initiate prompt intervention in time for an optimal outcome. The classic presentation of acute postoperative bacterial endophthalmitis includes a red and painful eye associated with frequent headaches and prominent visual loss during the second to the seventh day after surgery. The rapidly progressive symptoms are accompanied by diffuse lid and corneal edema, conjunctival discharge, as well as anterior chamber and vitreous infiltrates. The increasing intraocular proteinaceous infiltrates frequently result in the layering of a fibrin clot within the bottom of the anterior chamber, known as a hypopyon. Invasion of the retina and optic nerve by the infecting organism invariably leads to progressive disc and retinal edema and hemorrhage, posterior fibrin deposits, as well as tissue necrosis. The eventual severe retinal destruction results in profound visual loss. The necrotic retina is also prone to develop retinal breaks and detachments during and subsequent to the course of the endophthalmitis. Whether other clinical features are present or not, the cardinal sign and the only consistent and reliable indicator of postoperative endophthalmitis is unexplained vitreous inflammation and opacification. In the Endophthalmitis Vitrectomy Study (EVS), pain was absent in 25% of cases and hypopyon was lacking in 14% of cases. Typical clinical signs may also be masked and their onset delayed on account of postoperative antibiotic and corticosteroid usage, as well as the low virulence of the causative organism.

ORGANISMS ASSOCIATED WITH ACUTE POSTOPERATIVE ENDOPHTHALMITIS

The most common microbial isolate from acute postoperative endophthalmitis is a gram-positive organism; specifically, a coagulase-negative *Staphylococcus*. The EVS reported 70% of the isolates to be coagulase-negative micrococci (predominantly staphylococci). Twenty-four point two percentage (24.2%) of the isolates consisted of other gram-positive organisms as follow: 9.9% *Staphylococcus aureus*, 9.0% *Streptococcus* species, 2.2% *Enterococcus* species, and 3.1% miscellaneous gram-positive species (0.6% *Propionibacterium* species, 1.2% *Corynebacterium* species, 0.6% *Bacillus* species, and 0.6% *Diphtheroid*). Gram-negative organisms were isolated in 5.9% of the cases in the EVS (1.9% *Proteus mirabilis*, 1.2% *Pseudomonas* species, 0.6% *Morganella morganii*, 0.6% *Citrobacter diversus*, 0.3% *Serratia marcescens*, 0.6% *Enterobacter* species, and 0.3% *Flavobacterium* species). It is possible that the EVS may have underestimated the rate of gram-negative infection for postoperative endophthalmitis by excluding eyes with corneal opacities severe enough to preclude a vitrectomy. Table 3.1 outlines a typical spectrum of microbial isolates associated with acute postoperative endophthalmitis (reported in the EVS), as well as distinctive spectra of microbial isolates associated with other types of endophthalmitis.

DELAYED-ONSET ENDOPHTHALMITIS

Chronic or late-onset endophthalmitis is defined as the presentation of indolent intraocular inflammation one or more months after ocular surgery. Traditionally, fungal endophthalmitis has often been cited as an example of late-onset endophthalmitis. However, recent reports have also implicated other organisms associated with this category of endophthalmitis. In their review of 19 cases of delayed-onset pseudophakic endophthalmitis, Fox and associates reported 63% of those cases to be due to *Propionibacterium acnes*, 16% to *Candida parapsilosis*, 16% to *Staphylococcus epidermidis*, and 5% to *Corynebacterium* species. Ficker et al. isolated *Staphylococcus epidermidis* and *Achromobacter* species from eyes with chronic bacterial endophthalmitis.

PROPIONIBACTERIUM ENDOPHTHALMITIS

In 1986, Meister and associates described the syndrome of *Propionibacterium acnes* endophthalmitis with delayed onset after extracapsular cataract extraction (ECCE) with posterior chamber intraocular lens (PCIOL) implantation. *Propionibacterium* is a gram-positive, nonspore-forming, pleomorphic and anaerobic bacillus. It is ubiquitous in nature and a common component of the bacterial flora of the ocular and periocular tissues, including the conjunctiva and the sebaceous follicles. It is an opportunistic pathogen frequently associated with a low-grade, delayed-onset, and persistent endophthalmitis after cataract extraction with an intraocular implant. The typical clinical presentation may include an indolent course of chronic low-grade iridocyclitis with one or more of the following signs: large white granulomatous or nongranulomatous keratic precipitates, hypopyon, beaded fibrin strands in the anterior chamber, vitritis, intraretinal hemorrhages and infiltrates, and a prominent whitish plaque on the residual lens capsule. The last feature is considered to be a hallmark sign of *P. acnes* endophthalmitis. Previous biopsies of lens capsules with the whitish exudates have yielded *P. acnes* on histological studies and cultures, proving that they contain foci of sequestered *P. acnes* organisms. The delayed activation and proliferation of the sequestered organisms result in a chronic and indolent course of endophthalmitis. Since *P. acnes* is a low virulent and fastidious bacillus, it is difficult to isolate and grow in culture. Specimens of suspected cases of *P. acnes* endophthalmitis should be promptly inoculated into anaerobic media. *P. acnes* may not appear in culture until 5 days or more after inoculation. It has been pointed out that the *P. acnes* organisms isolated from eyes with acute postoperative endophthalmitis may constitute a less resilient form than those from eyes with the delayed-onset or chronic type of endophthalmitis. Unlike the chronic *P. acnes* infection, the acute type is usually easily eradicated with intravitreal antibiotic injections alone and has a low recurrence rate. In contrast, the chronic *P. acnes* endophthalmitis frequently requires a vitrectomy and capsulectomy to eliminate the sequestered organisms.

DIAGNOSTIC WORKUP AND MICROBIOLOGICAL STUDIES

When managing an eye with suspected endophthalmitis, the clinician must first perform a careful evaluation. It is important to pay close attention to certain ocular features that may modify the course and influence the management of the infection: e.g. wound leak and dehiscence, iris and vitreous prolapse, flat anterior chamber, corneal and suture abscess, bleb defects, eroding scleral suture associated with a sutured posterior chamber implant, etc. A successful outcome entails the correction of the above abnormalities besides effective antimicrobial therapy. One must also differentiate endophthalmitis from other conditions with similar clinical features, such as a corneal ulcer and aseptic anterior uveitis with a hypopyon, and vitreous infiltration due to sterile posterior uveitis or retained lens fragments, phacoanaphylactic uveitis, etc. In addition, a search for concomitant conditions that may complicate the course of the endophthalmitis is an important part of the workup, e.g. superimposed retinal breaks or detachment, choroidal detachment, located lens fragments, and intraocular foreign body, etc. Ancillary diagnostic tools such as ultrasonography may contribute to the diagnostic workup.

TECHNIQUES OF SPECIMEN COLLECTION

Aqueous and vitreous specimens may be obtained in an office setting or at the time of a vitrectomy. In the former situation, careful administration of local anesthesia (topical, subconjunctival, peribulbar, or retrobulbar) and sterile prepping with 5% povidone-iodine solution are recommended. A small volume of aqueous specimen (0.1 to 0.2 mL) is then carefully withdrawn via a 27- or 30-gauge needle at the limbus into a tuberculin syringe. The vitreous specimen may be obtained with one of the following two methods: **(A) Needle tap:** A 22- to 27-gauge needle attached to a tuberculin syringe is inserted through the pars plana into the vitreous cavity for gentle aspiration of 0.1 to 0.3 mL of liquid vitreous. Excessive force must be avoided to prevent vitreoretinal traction. A "dry tap" requires the conversion to a mechanized biopsy. **(B) Mechanized vitreous biopsy:** A one-, two-, or three- port pars plana vitrectomy with a mechanized 20-gauge vitrectomy probe is employed for the biopsy. A small volume of undiluted specimen (up to 0.3 mL) from the anterior vitreous is collected into a sterile syringe connected to the aspiration line of the vitrectomy probe through gentle manual suction by a surgical assistant during the vitrectomy. Diluted specimens collected into a larger syringe or into a vitrectomy cassette may also be concentrated either with the suction filtered technique or the centrifuged method (Fig. 3.13A to C). The former involves passing the diluted specimens in an upper sterile chamber through a membrane filter with 0.45-micron pores into a lower chamber connected to suction. With the aid of sterile forceps and scissors or knives, the membrane filter containing the concentrated specimens is then cut into small pieces for direct inoculation on solid and into liquid media for cultures (Fig. 3.13). Concentrated specimens scraped off the surface of the membrane filter are also applied on slides for preparation of various stains. The alternative centrifuged method requires the transfer of the diluted specimens into a sterile centrifuge tube for high-speed centrifuge. The sediments from the centrifuged tube are then processed for microbiological stains and cultures (Fig. 3.13). In 1993, Donahue and associates reported a significant increase in positive yield with culturing the contents of a vitrectomy cassette after concentration of the specimen in comparison to culturing the specimen from a needle tap or a limited mechanized vitreous biopsy (76% versus 43%). In the EVS, some degree of culture growth was achieved from 82.8% of the tested vitrectomy cassette specimens, and the vitrectomy cassette fluid was the only source of a positive culture for 8.9% of eyes. The EVS found that the vitrectomy cassette specimen had prognostic significance equivalent to growth from other intraocular sources.

ENDOPHTHALMITIS
(ANTERIOR CHAMBER WASHOUT BEFORE VITRECTOMY)

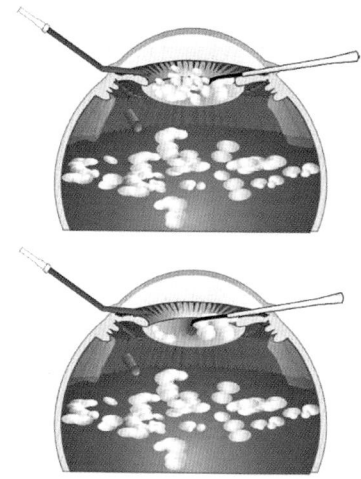

Fig. 3.14 Endophthalmitis (anterior chamber washout before vitrectomy) (*Courtesy*: Clement Chan)

The technique of eliminating cloudy fibrin deposits, membranes, and hyphema from the anterior chamber is illustrated. A microsurgical hook or pick inserted at the limbus is used to scrape off the cloudy material from the IOL and iris surface before removing them with a vitrectomy probe from the anterior chamber. A separate probe also inserted at the limbus for anterior chamber infusion is often necessary to prevent chamber collapse. The posterior infusion fluid is not turned on until adequate media clarity is achieved to ascertain the proper location of the tip of the posterior infusion cannula.

The two fundamental therapeutic modalities for treating infectious endophthalmitis in the modern world comprise of antimicrobial therapy and vitrectomy (Fig. 3.14). When appropriate, they may be supplemented with anti-inflammatory therapy for reducing damages induced by the infection. Applying effective strategies for antimicrobial therapy constitutes the most critical aspect of the management of endophthalmitis.

ANTIMICROBIAL THERAPY

Topical and Subconjunctival

Prophylactic Therapy

Multiple studies have demonstrated that preoperative application of antiseptics and antibiotics with a broad-spectrum antimicrobial coverage reduces the eyelid and conjunctival bacterial counts, resulting in decreased potential for postoperative endophthalmitis. Apt and associates reported that a single preoperative application of half-strength (5%) povidone-iodine solution in the conjunctival cul-de-sac was equivalent to a 3-day course of prophylactic topical combination solution of neomycin sulfate, polymyxin B sulfate, and gramicidin in reducing the bacterial colonies.

Therapy after the Onset of Endophthalmitis

With the exception of mild infections, topical and subconjunctival drug delivery usually constitutes only adjunctive antimicrobial therapy after the onset of endophthalmitis. However, they are essential for certain conditions that may accompany the endophthalmitis (i.e. bleb infection, corneal ulcer, wound or suture abscess, etc.) A typical regimen of supplemental topical therapy for acute postoperative bacterial endophthalmitis includes frequent application of antibiotics with appropriate antibacterial coverage, as well as repeated administration of anti-inflammatory and cycloplegic drugs. Steroid is avoided for fungal cases. The use of customized fortified doses of topical antimicrobial drugs (e.g. 45 to 50 mg per mL of vancomycin, 50 mg per mL of cefazolin, cefamandole or ceftazidime, 50 mg per mL of ampicillin, 50 mg per mL of clindamycin, 1% solution of methicillin, 8 to 15 mg per mL of tobramycin, 10 to 20 mg per mL of gentamicin or amikacin, 0.15 to 0.5% of amphotericin B, or 10 mg per mL of miconazole, etc.) has been a common practice in the course of treating the endophthalmitis. However, the potential benefit of the fortified doses over the regular doses remains controversial and unproven. Another common practice is supplemental subconjunctival therapy (e.g. 25 mg of vancomycin, 100 to 125 mg of cefazolin, or ceftazidime, 75 mg of cefamandole, 100 mg of ampicillin or methicillin, 20 to 40 mg of gentamicin, tobramycin or amikacin, 30 mg of clindamycin, or 5 mg of miconazole). The degree of synergy between subconjunctival and intravitreal antimicrobial therapy is unknown.

Intravitreal Antimicrobial Therapy

For all categories of endophthalmitis besides the endogenous type, the mainstay of therapy is prompt and direct intravitreal injections of antimicrobial drugs. It is imperative that the intravitreal antimicrobial therapy first provides comprehensive coverage for the gram-positive organisms, since they constitute the majority of the microbial isolates associated with endophthalmitis (94% in the EVS).

The following antibiotic combinations are the current recommended initial empiric intravitreal antibiotic regimens for acute postoperative bacterial endophthalmitis in a clinical setting:
- Vancomycin 1.0 mg/0.1 mL and ceftazidime 2.25 mg/0.1 mL; or
- Vancomycin 1.0 mg/0.1 mL and amikacin (100 to 400 micrograms/0.1 mL) for beta-lactam sensitive patients.

Systemic Antimicrobial Therapy

Although the EVS found systemic antimicrobial therapy provide no additional benefit to intravitreal therapy for acute postoperative endophthalmitis, its role for other types of endophthalmitis is more important. Concomitant intravitreal and systemic antibiotic therapy besides vitrectomy remains to be the standard of care (based on clinical experience but without experimental support) for most bleb-related and trauma-induced endophthalmitis. For endogenous endophthalmitis, appropriate systemic (especially intravenous) therapy with maximal doses for intravitreal penetration is the key for a successful outcome. Intravenous antibiotic therapy is generally required for two weeks for most endogenous cases, and as long as four or more weeks for endocarditis cases.

CORTICOSTEROID THERAPY

The use of intravitreal corticosteroids for non-fungal endophthalmitis remains controversial due to a lack of randomized controlled studies. The potential benefits of corticosteroid therapy for endophthalmitis include inhibition of macrophage and neutrophil migration, stabilization of lysosomal membranes resulting in decreased degranulation of inflammatory cells (neutrophils, mast cells, macrophages, basophils), and reduction in prostaglandin synthesis and capillary permeability due to inhibition of phospholipase A_2. However, its potential harmful effects and limitations include possible reduction in the killing power of inflammatory cells, changes in the bioavailability and doses of the intravitreal antibiotics, potentiation of the infection in the absence of appropriate antibiotic therapy, risk of retinal toxicity due to medication errors, and inability to counteract bacterial toxin-induced damages. The standard clinical dose of intravitreal dexamethasone is 400 micrograms per 0.1 mL, although the optimal dose has not been determined. Besides intravitreal injections, other routes of steroid therapy include subconjunctival injections (4 to 12 mg of dexamethasone or 40 mg of triamcinolone or depomedrol) and systemic therapy (1 mg/kg/day for 5 days followed by rapid tapering). When fungal endophthalmitis is suspected, most authorities advocate the avoidance of corticosteroid.

VITRECTOMY

Indications for Vitrectomy

The theoretical advantages of vitrectomy include the removal of infectious organisms with their toxins and inflammatory mediators, clearing of vitreous opacities and sequestered abscess pockets, collection of abundant specimens for cultures, elimination of vitreous membranes to avoid vitreoretinal traction, allowing increased space for intraocular drug administration, and possible improved diffusion of intravitreal antibiotics. For chronic endophthalmitis due to the *Propionibacterium* species, intravitreal antibiotics alone may not be sufficient. Frequently, a vitrectomy combined with a partial or complete removal of the lens capsule with sequestered organisms (sometimes including the implant), is required for a successful outcome.

Vitrectomy Techniques

A three-port pars plana vitrectomy using standard 20-gauge instruments and concentrating on the "core" vitreous is usually recommended, although a one- or two-port approach may be sufficient for a limited vitreous biopsy. A portable battery-driven 23-gauge vitrector is also commercially available for a limited vitreous biopsy. The greater potential for surgical complications associated with increased tissue vulnerability induced by the endophthalmitis requires the surgeon to be well versed with vitreoretinal techniques and vigilant throughout the vitrectomy. The use of a long infusion cannula (e.g. 6 mm) is often advantageous in preventing subretinal and choroidal infusion for pseudophakic eyes and post-traumatic eyes requiring a lensectomy, in light of multiple predisposing factors for such a complication with endophthalmitis (e.g. limited intraocular tissue visibility, increased choroidal congestion, frequent hypotony, etc.) To further avoid such a complication, the surgeon must ensure that the tip of the infusion cannula is well within the vitreous cavity before turning on the infusion fluid. For a case with very cloudy media, the surgeon may confirm this by gently rubbing the tip of a microvitreoretinal blade inserted through one of the superior sclerotomies against the tip of the infusion cannula. Frequently, a separate anterior chamber washout via a limbal approach is required to eliminate cloudy fibrin deposits and hyphema from the anterior chamber initially, before sufficient anterior media clarity is attained for a pars plana vitrectomy. Various microsurgical hooks and picks may be inserted through the limbus to scrape off the anterior chamber infiltrates or membranes layered on the surface of the implant and the iris before removing them with a vitrectomy probe from the anterior chamber (Fig. 3.14). A separate anterior infusion line may be required during the anterior chamber washout to prevent chamber collapse. When performing a core vitrectomy, care must be taken to apply only gentle intraocular movements and avoid vigorous surgical maneuvers that may induce vitreoretinal traction, such as aggressive epiretinal membrane retrieval and fibrin clean up. Despite the intentional avoidance of their direct removal during the vitrectomy, the posterior epiretinal fibrin deposits and dense retinal hemorrhages tend to gradually dissolve following the injections of intravitreal antimicrobial and anti-inflammatory medications after surgery. Keeping the intraocular instruments well within the anterior and central vitreous cavity and staying away from the fragile infected retina during surgery will reduce the chance of retinal complications. Vitreous specimen for microbial investigation is either collected into a syringe connected to the aspiration line of the vitrectomy probe or into a cassette of the vitrectomy machine Finally, the eye is made sufficiently soft to allow space for injections of medications and the sclerotomies are closed tightly to avoid fluid leaks, before the administration of intravitreal drugs at the end of the surgery.

CYSTOID MACULAR EDEMA

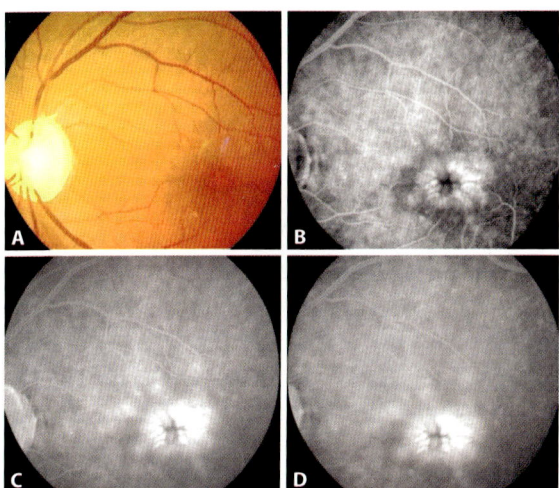

Figs 3.15A to D Fundus photograph and fluorescein angiography depicting CME. (A) Color fundus photograph of cystoid macular edema; (B to D) Fundus fluorescein photograph of cystoid macular edema (flower petal appearance); (B) Shows capillary leakage in the macular area; (C) Early flower petal appearance; (D) Late flower petal appearance

Since its recognition as a distinct entity by Irvine in 1953 and its elaborate clinical description by Gass and Norton in 1966, aphakic and pseudophakic cystoid macular edema, commonly referred to as the Irvine Gass syndrome, has continued to perplex ophthalmologists in terms of its pathogenesis, its peculiar clinical manifestations and its treatment. It is one of the most frequent and troublesome problems following cataract surgery with or without IOL.

MACULAR EDEMA

The extracellular space of the retina normally constitutes a small proportion of its total volume. Active transport of electrolytes and larger molecules from the retina across the retinal pigment epithelium to the blood maintains this situation. Disruption of either the inner or outer blood-retinal barrier leads to leakage of plasma proteins and water, which leads to expansion of the extra cellular fluid space of the retina. This is often accompanied by accumulation of fluid in the macular area, especially in the outer plexiform layer and inner nuclear layer. Retinal edema localized to the macula is called macular edema. More generalized leakage leads to diffuse thickening of the posterior pole. Accumulation of fluid in cystic spaces leads to cystoid macular edema.

CYSTOID MACULAR EDEMA

The reason why the macula is the most commonly involved part of the retina is because of its peculiar anatomy characterized by abundance of axons (Nerve fiber layer of Henle), paucity of glial tissue which holds the retinal elements together, relative lack of vasculature and greater metabolic activity.

Theories Explaining Aphakic and Pseudophakic CME

Vitreous Traction Theory

Constant constriction and dilatation of the pupil creates pulling on the anterior vitreous strands, which is transmitted to the vitreous base and thence to the macula by presumed vitreous connections between the posterior hyaloid and the surface of the macula. This is the vitreous Tug syndrome. Vitreoretinal adhesion is strongest at those regions where the internal limiting lamina is thinnest, i.e the fovea and vitreous base. In these regions, the Muller cell attachment plaques to the Internal limiting membrane are most prominent. Thus it appears that the continuity of structure between the collagen fibrils of the vitreous and the Muller cells of the retina could directly transmit any movement, displacement or traction in the vitreous to the Muller cells of the macula. Since Muller cells are not only trans-retinal structural elements but also serve a vital metabolic role, any damage to these cells could alter other components of the macula. Chronic Müller cell irritation may also lead to the local release of a variety of mediators, which in turn facilitates leakage.

Inflammation Theory

Eyes with CME nearly always demonstrate signs of intra ocular inflammation and also respond to steroid therapy. Clinical observations associating aphakic CME with intraocular inflammation have been made for many years. Aqueous humor contains biochemically active principles called Aqueous Biotoxic Complex (ABC) factors, which manifest biotoxic effects when it leaves its natural reservoir. If large amounts of it are produced or if there is a reduction in its absorption by the ciliary epithelium, these diffuse posteriorly through the collapsed liquefied vitreous gel. The liquefied vitreous anterior to the retina hence assumes chemical and osmotic properties quite unlike those normally present, which results in an outpouring of fluid from the perimacular capillaries. The lower incidence of CME after ECCE may be due to the presence of an intact posterior capsule, which acts as a diffusion barrier. The ABC factors may be prostaglandins, which are synthesized de novo. Since the eye does not contain the enzyme 15-PG dehydrogenase to deactivate prostaglandins their removal is dependant on an active transport pump called the Bito's pump located in the ciliary epithelium. This pump is inoperable (overburdened or inhibited) for at least three weeks after ocular trauma. The inflammatory state persists for longer periods when vitreous is adherent to the cataract wound causing pupillary distortion.

Anoxia Theory

This is not yet proved. An association between CME and systemic conditions, e.g. Hypertension, arteriosclerotic heart disease and diabetes mellitus is seen in which anoxia could be predisposing factor for CME.

Theories Concerning the Origin of Cysts of CME

Intracellular Theory

Yanoff et al. and Fine and Brucker proposed that cysts develop from degenerating Müller's cells. Initially these cells demonstrate oedema, which gradually increases until the cytoplasm of the cells begin to develop vacuoles. The edematous cells gradually expand until the cell walls break and adjoining cells from larger cavities leading to the cysts in CME. A breakdown of the blood-retinal barrier or anoxia is the primary cause of the edema.

Extracellular Theory

Gass, Anderson and Davis proposed that cysts arise from expansion of the extra cellular spaces of the retina by serous exudation within the outer plexiform layer and inner nuclear layer. This involves leakage of serous exudates from perifoveal intraretinal capillaries and sometimes from disc capillaries. The exudates form small puddles in the OPL of Henle which acts like a sponge because of the peculiar structure of the macula. This theory is supported by the highly reversible function of a CME eye which argues against cellular death and disruption and also the visible lack of occluded capillaries in the macula which argues against the presence of anoxia.

CME AND ACIOL—POSSIBLE PATHOPHYSIOLOGY

Chronic anterior uveal irritation may either stimulate production of intra ocular inflammatory substances or may retard the absorption or removal of these substances by the non-pigmented epithelium of the ciliary body. An ACIOL which can press against the anterior surface of the iris or apply constant pressure on the face of the ciliary body could trigger constant anterior uveal inflammation. Older style IOL's situated with in the pupil (intracameral) that either rest upon the pupillary margin or have haptics sutured to the iris stroma possess the same, if not greater propensity to elicit chronic uveal irritation. Hence, intracameral and ACIOL's are more likely to stimulate CME than are PCIOL's.

Incidence of CME

Irvine originally reported an incidence of 2% but the incidence of angiographic CME is much higher, occurring approximately after 40% of intracapsular cataract extractions. Also if it occurs in one eye, there is almost a 70% probability of it affecting the second eye as well after cataract surgery. Phacoemulsification with "in the bag" IOL placement has been reported to have an incidence as low as 0.5%. Eyes with a primary posterior capsulotomy had a significantly higher incidence of angiographic CME approximately 21.5% as compared to 5.6% in eyes with intact capsules in one series whereas in another series no statistically significant difference was found in the incidence of angiographic CME 6 weeks or 6 months postoperatively. The incidence of clinically significant pseudophakic CME after Nd: YAG laser posterior capsulotomy was around 1.23% in one study.

CLINICAL APPEARANCE OF CME

Slit Lamp Examination

This is done with Hruby Lens, 90 D Lens, 78 D Lens or the Goldmann 3 mirror contact lens. Advantages are the use of slit lamp optics and stereopsis. Biomicroscopic examination with Hruby lens or a fundus contact lens or a 90 D lens shows a characteristic honey comb lesion with one or more larger cystoid spaces centrally and any number of smaller, oval spaces around them. Cystoid spaces are best seen using red free light, which makes the inner walls visible. The optical section of the convex anterior walls of the cysts can be seen overlying optically empty vesicles, tightly packed together with their interfaces presenting a spidery pattern. With the slit beam, it is possible to see a network of interlacing, fine refractile lines by retroillumination. The retina may be markedly thickened and the lesion may be as large as 1.5–2 disk diameters. Some cases may be associated with discedema.

Direct Ophthalmoscopy

This usually shows a loss of foveal reflex. Monochromatic light is better for detecting subtle macular changes hence red free light can be used. Using the macular aperture, the beam is passed slowly back and forth across the macula. The septa may be observed by retroillumination, i.e. just adjacent to the edge of the light beam. Disadvantages are the lack of stereoscopic view and the difficulty of recoding and transmitting information.

Indirect Ophthalmoscopy

This is useful in ruling out other causes of CME.

Anterior Segment Examination

This usually shows signs of inflammation. The anterior hyaloid face may be intact or broken and the vitreous usually shows cells and vitreous opacities and posterior vitreous detachment.

Fundus Fluorescein Angiography

This is used to confirm and document macular changes and for deciding the management and also for follow-up. In CME, within one to two minutes of dye injection, leakage into the macula is seen (Figs 3.15A to D). A stellate pattern with feathery margins is seen by 5–15 minutes usually, but sometimes taking upto 30 minutes. The pattern seen on FFA is called the flower petal appearance. The dark septae in the macular area that compartmentalize the pattern are because of the Müller's fibers. The spaces appear to intercommunicate. Usually there is considerable leakage of dye into the vitreous and aqueous anteriorly. In some patients with disc edema, there may be leakage of dye into the optic nerve and peripapillary retina.

Various FFA grading systems have been used for CME:
Grade 0: No edema
Grade 1+: Capillary leakage
Grade 2+: Partial petaloid ring
Grade 3+: Complete petaloid ring
Level 1: Edema less than perifoveal
Level 2: Minimal perifoveal edema
Level 3: Moderate perifoveal edema (1 DD)
Level 4: Severe perifoveal edema.

OPTICAL COHERENCE TOMOGRAPHY IN CME

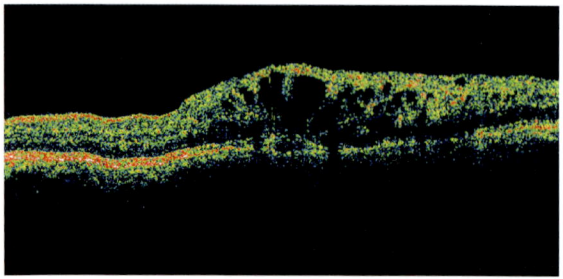

Fig. 3.16 Depicting CME

MACULAR FUNCTION TESTS IN CYSTOID MACULAR EDEMA

Best corrected visual acuity and visual acuity with pin hole, two point discrimination, Maddox Rod test, all indicate decreased macular function. Amsler grid chart may show central distortion of the grids or a relative central scotoma. The automated perimeter has special macular programs, which may show central scotoma. Any blanks or scotoma in the central area on entoptic imagery implies macular involvement. Potential Acuity Meter (PAM) can be used for differentiating between visual loss from anterior segment disease and macular disease. Longer recovery time, up to 90–180 seconds on macular photostress test implies macular dysfunction even though the area may appear anatomically normal. The normal recovery time is 55 seconds. Difference between the two eyes is also significant.

In cases of opaque media, the visual acuity can be determined with clinical interferometers. Electrophysiology may also show changes in CME. Foveal ERG is a test of the temporal responsiveness of the central 10 degree of the retina and requires integrity of the outer retinal layers, especially Müller's cells. FERG is usually abnormal in 35% of CME eyes. Pattern ERG reflects the inner retinal layer function. It is usually abnormal in 53% of CME eyes. Over half of the PERG abnormal eyes had no associated FERG abnormalities. OCT should also be done in cases of CME (Fig. 3.16).

SEQUELA OF CME: POST-CME LAMELLAR HOLE

Permanent macular degeneration may arise secondary to prolonged chronic CME. The cystoid spaces of the macula may coalesce together so that all retinal elements disappear except for the internal limiting membrane. After the internal limiting membrane also disintegrates, a lamellar hole is formed which may be one-fourth to one-third disc diameter in size. Surrounding intact cystoid spaces may be seen. In the presence of a lamellar hole visual acuity may continue to be good because of the retention of some percipient elements. Rarely does CME progress to a full thickness macular hole.

On-Off Phenomenon

The CME tends to be cyclic in nature, so that sometimes on withdrawing treatment following good response to therapy, CME may relapse again which is called the on-off phenomenon.

PROPHYLACTIC TREATMENT

- Steady and gentle preoperative ocular compression.
- Avoiding ICCE and unplanned ECCE.
- Gentle tissue handling and avoiding excessive instrumentation.
- Avoiding complications like posterior capsular rent, vitreous loss, iris prolapse, etc.
- Proper management of vitreous loss with thorough anterior vitrectomy.
- In the bag IOL placement.
- IOL with chemically inert haptics and high quality optics with good surface finish and correct dimensions.
- Avoiding photoxicity by using coaxial light only when red reflex is essential and using oblique illumination at all other times. Also by using a pupil occluder, decreasing the intensity of illumination and by rotating the macula away from light during suturing and also by using an IOL with UV absorbing optics.
- Pharmacological prophylaxis with postoperative steroids and nonsteroidal anti-inflammatory drugs (NSAIDs) through

topical, subconjunctival, sub-tenon or systemic routes. The use of steroids and NSAIDs decreases the amount of intraocular inflammatory substances released at the time of surgery.

THERAPY FOR ESTABLISHED CME

Medical Therapy

- *Topical steroids*: They are given 4–6 times per day.
- *Repository steroid injections*: Methylprednisolone acetate suspension (Depo-Medrol) or triamcinolone acetonide (Kenalog), usually 40 mg (1 mL) is given subconjunctivally once a month. It is not to be used in eyes with a known propensity for steroid induced rise in IOP.
- *Systemic steroids*: Efficacy is not known as yet. Dosage: 40–100 mg per day or every alternate day.
- *Topical NSAIDs*: Topical indomethacin 1%, Ketorolac 0.5% Diclofenac 0.1% and Flurbiprofen 0.03% can be tried. Studies have shown an improvement in vision but an on-off phenomenon may be seen.
- *Oral NSAID therapy*: Indomethacin 25 mg tid after meals can be tried. Other drugs are suprofen, fenoprofen, ibuprofen, piroxicam. All these can cause gastric irritation.
- *Hyperbaric oxygen*: Some patients receiving 2.2 atm, oxygen for 1.5 hours twice daily for 7 days and then 2 hours daily for 14 days may show improvement. Hyperbaric oxygen may

help heal injured capillary complexes by causing constriction of the macular capillaries along with stimulating collagen formation, which seals these spaces.

- *Acetazolamide*: It facilitates transport of water across the RPE from the subretinal space to the choroid. Dosage is 250–500 mg bid or qid.

Medical therapy can also be tried for many elderly patients and for unwilling patients who do not want further surgery.

ND-YAG Laser Vitreolysis

This avoids an invasive procedure. Elevated vitreous strands are transected using Nd-YAG laser. Bisecting vitreous membranes that are adherent to the anterior surface of the iris may be difficult without producing small hemorrhages which diffuse into the aqueous and make accurate focusing impossible. Therefore laser treatment is primarily used in those cases in which vitreous strands bridge the margin of the pupil to the undersurface of the cataract wound without adhering to the anterior surface of the iris.

Surgical Therapy

For Aphakic CME

Vitrectomy: The goal of the surgery is to remove all formed vitreous elements from the anterior segment to restore the anatomy of the iris and pupil to a state as near normal as possible. Technique—the edges of the condensed sheets of solid vitreous adherent to the anterior surface of the iris are carefully identified with the slit lamp preoperatively and with the operating microscope intraoperatively. Then a plane of dissection is created between the sheet of vitreous and the anterior surface of the iris by the to and fro swings of a microcyclodialysis spatula introduced at 90° to the edge. The sheet is then removed by advancing a vitrectomy instrument beneath it. This is done till all formed vitreous is removed and the pupil is restored to normal. Next, a shallow vitrectomy is performed at the level of the pupil to prevent new strands of vitreous from finding their way to the incision site postoperatively. If a pars plana approach is used, a complete posterior vitrectomy can also be done.

For Pseudophakic CME with ACIOL

- With relatively round pupil: Removal of the ACIOL with anterior vitrectomy is done. The surgical aphakia is corrected either with a sulcus IOL if adequate posterior capsular rim remains (but the disadvantage here is irritation to the uveal tissue) or a scleral fixated IOL. Other solutions are contact lenses, epikeratoplasty, Excimer laser, or peripheral intrastromal corneal ring.
- With moderate pupillary distortion from disrupted vitreous or malpositioned haptics: Anterior vitrectomy and anterior

segment restoration is done. The IOL may be left in situ or exchanged.

For Pseudophakic CME with PCIOL

- With pupillary distortion: Anterior segment restoration with a core pars plana vitrectomy is done.
- With in-the-bag IOL, intact posterior capsule, normal mobile pupil, no peripheral anterior synechiae: Here a pars plana vitrectomy could be performed to remove the vitreous sump or vitreous traction from the macula, but the sump theory is not yet proved, hence it is better not to operate. If done to release vitreomacular traction, such traction should be confirmed preoperatively by biomicroscopic examination with posterior pole contact lens. This situation is rare and hence surgical intervention should be uncommon. But before resorting to surgery in such cases, other causes for CME should be ruled out and a complete course of medical therapy should have been tried.

GLUED IOL

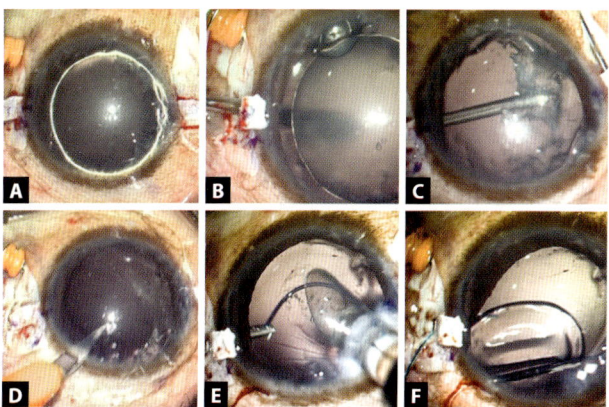

Figs 3.17A to F Glued IOL being done in a case of spherophakia with anterior dislocation of crystalline lens. (A) Two partial thickness scleral flaps made 180° opposite to each other; (B) Sclerotomy being done with a 20 G needle about 1.5 mm away from the limbus beneath the scleral flaps; (C) Lensectomy with vitrectomy done with a 23 G vitrectomy probe introduced from the sclerotomy site; (D) A side port incision is framed midway between the left sclerotomy site and the central corneal tunnel; (E) A 3-piece foldable IOL is injected and the tip of the haptic is grasped with a glued IOL forceps; (F) After the IOL unfolds, the leading haptic is externalized

Glued IOL is a type of secondary IOL fixation that helps to fix an IOL without an element of pseudophakodonesis in the eye. It has a wide array of application and it can be clubbed with various surgeries that necessitate a secondary IOL implantation in the eye. Two partial thickness scleral flaps are made 180° opposite to each other (Fig. 3.17A). Sclerotomy is done with a 20 G needle about 1–1.5 mm behind the limbus beneath the flaps (Fig. 3.17B). Vitrectomy is then performed with a 23 G cutter introduced from the sclerotomy site (Fig. 3.17C). A side port incision is framed midway between the left sclerotomy and the corneal section (Fig. 3.17D). A 3-piece foldable IOL is loaded on to the cartridge and is introduced into the eye. The tip of the leading haptic is grasped with a glued IOL forceps (Fig. 3.17E) introduced from the left sclerotomy site. Once the entire IOL has unfolded, the haptic is pulled and externalized (Fig. 3.17F).

GLUED IOL (CONTINUED)

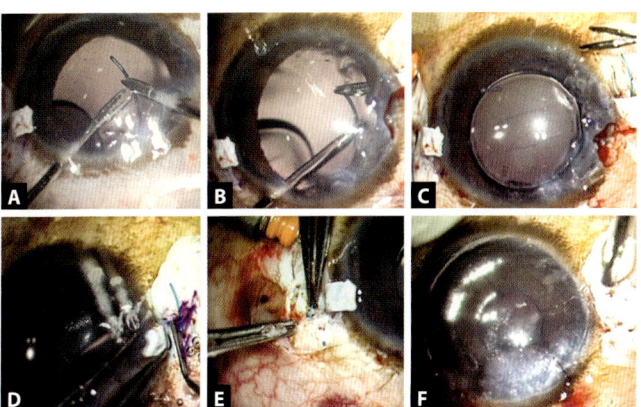

Figs 3.18A to F Glued IOL procedure (continued). (A) The trailing haptic is flexed in to the eye and 'Handshake technique' is performed; (B) Tip of the trailing haptic with the glued IOL forceps introduced from the right sclerotomy site; (C) Both haptics are externalized; (D) Scleral pocket being created with a 26 G needle along the edge of the base of the flap; parallel to the sclerotomy site; (E) Haptics are tucked in to the scleral pockets; (F) Infusion is stopped and fibrin glue is applied beneath the flaps to seal the wound and the conjunctival incision too

The trailing haptic is then flexed into the eye and the haptic is transferred to the glued IOL forceps introduced from the side port incision (Fig. 3.18A). The forceps in the right hand is withdrawn and is re-introduced from the right sclerotomy site (Fig. 3.18B). The trailing haptic is then transferred from the left to the right hand. This technique is known as 'Handshake technique'. The tip of the trailing haptic is grasped and both the haptics are then externalized (Fig. 3.18C). Scleral pockets are created with a 26 G needle (Fig. 3.18D) and the haptics are tucked in to it (Fig. 3.18E). Vitrectomy is performed at the sclerotomy site and the infusion is stopped. Fibrin glue is then applied beneath the flaps and is used to seal the conjunctival peritomy incisions (Fig. 3.18F).

TRAUMATIC IRIDODIALYSIS

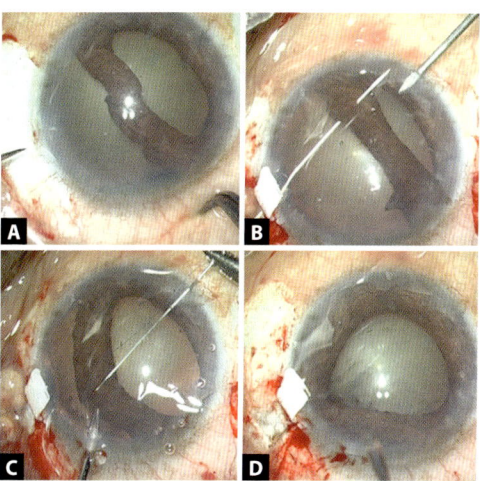

Figs 3.19A to D Iridodialysis repair. (A) Massive traumatic iridodialysis is depicted in the image; (B) A partial thickness scleral flap is made along the axis of maximum iridodialysis. A straight needle with 9-0 prolene suture is passed from peripheral end of the iris; (C) The needle exits the eye from the side port incision created on the opposite side by docking method. The needle is reintroduced into the eye from the same incision and is made to pass again from the peripheral part of the iris; (D) The suture is pulled and both the edges are tied together. This pulls the iris to the periphery and the pupil is reconstructed again

Blunt or penetrating trauma to the globe often damages the ocular structures and traumatic iridodialysis is an associated feature that a surgeon often comes across. The management of traumatic iridodialysis often depends upon its extent in clock hours and on its location. As depicted (Fig. 3.19A), massive iridodialysis is present that obstructs the visual axis. Such a scenario necessitates the surgical intervention.

A partial thickness scleral flap is created with its hinge towards the limbus along the axis of maximum iridodialysis. A straight needle with 9-0 prolene suture is passed from peripheral end of the iris (Fig. 3.19B) and by docking method this needle exits the eye from the side port incision created at the opposite end. The needle with attached suture re-enters the eye and is again passed from the peripheral base of the detached iris (Fig. 3.19C), close to the previous pass from the iris. The needle exits the eye from beneath the scleral flap and both the ends of the suture are tied with each other. The base of the iris is thus pulled in the periphery and reattaches (Fig. 3.19D).

BOSTON KERATOPROSTHESIS (KPro)

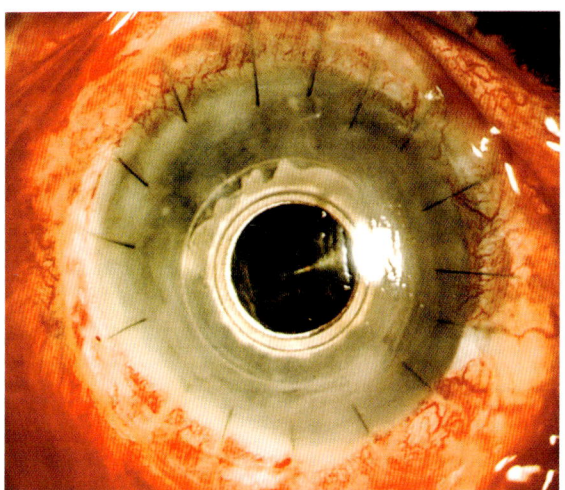

Fig. 3.20 Type-1 Boston Keratoprosthesis in place

The Boston Keratoprosthesis (KPro) (Fig. 3.20) is a type of artificial cornea and it is a treatment option for corneal disease that is not amenable to other standard corneal transplant procedure.

The Boston KPro is a collar button design prosthesis that is made up of three main components: a front plate with optical stem, a back plate and titanium locking c-ring. During assembly the front and back plates are snapped together with corneal tissue in between, which is then used to suture the device to the eye. It is available two types: Type I and Type II. Type I is the most commonly used type of prosthesis whereas Type II is reserved for severe end-stage ocular surface disease, and is similar to the type I device but requires a permanent tarsorrhaphy to be performed through which a small anterior nub of the type II model protrudes.

The indications for its use are multiple graft failure, Stevens-Johnson syndrome, ocular cicatricial pemphigoid, other autoimmune diseases, ocular burns and other conditions with poor prognosis with traditional penetrating keratoplasty.

Postoperatively, the procedure calls for lot of care and a regular follow-up of the patient as it can lead to devastating complications.

DECENTRATION OF THE CAPSULAR BAG AND IOL

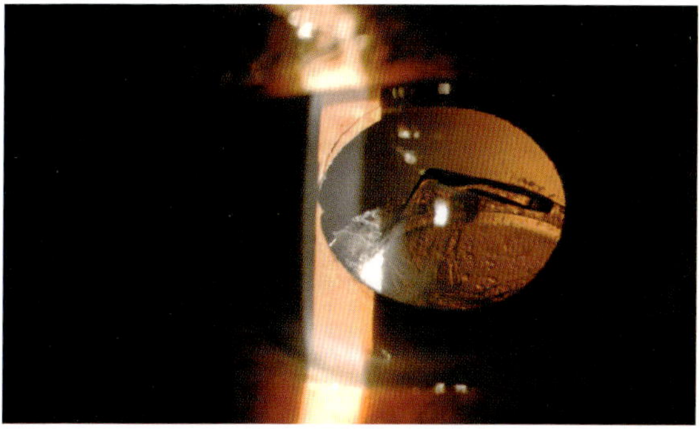

Fig. 3.21 Dislocated capsular bag IOL complex

Postoperative decentration of the capsular bag and the IOL can be seen in traumatic conditions or in zonulopathies as in systemic autoimmune disorders. The capsular bag and the IOL often need to be expelled from the eye followed by secondary IOL implant (Fig. 3.21).

Scleral tunnel incision can be framed and the bag-IOL complex is explanted from the eye. The tunnel is closed with a 10-0 nylon suture and an AC maintainer is introduced into the eye. Glued IOL procedure is then performed and the IOL is securely fixed followed by sealing of the scleral flaps and conjunctival opening with the help of glue.

If a 3-piece IOL is dislocated then the same IOL can be refixed into the eye without explanting it.

IOL SCAFFOLD

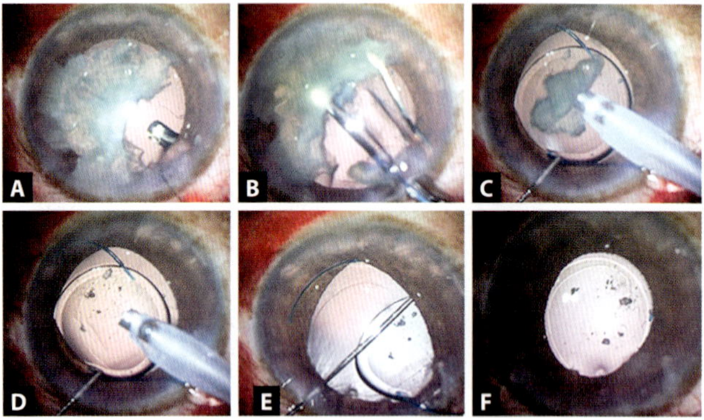

Figs 3.22A to F IOL scaffold. (A) Nuclear fragments levitated into the anterior chamber and pars plana vitrectomy is done to clear the vitreous from the pupillary axis; (B) A 3-piece foldable IOL being injected beneath the nuclear fragments; (C) The IOL is dialed by placing the haptics on to the surface of iris and the nuclear fragments are emulsified with the phaco probe. The IOL effectively compartmentalizes the eye and acts as a scaffold; (D) Nuclear fragments are completely emulsified; (E) IOL being dialed in the sulcus; (F) The IOL is well centered

Upon recognition of a PCR, dispersive viscoelastic is injected to seal the capsular break from the side port incision without withdrawal of the phaco probe. After adequate sealing of the rent, the phaco probe is withdrawn and dispersive OVD is used to levitate and bring all the nuclear remnants into the anterior chamber. In cases of small PCR's, the tear is converted into a posterior capsulorhexis; whereas in cases of large tears it is difficult to do so. A 23/25 G vitrectomy probe is introduced with high cutting rate and adequate suction parameters. The infusion needle can be used to maintain the anterior chamber during vitrectomy; care being taken so that the fluid does not push the nuclear fragments down. The direction of the flow should be beneath the nuclear fragment towards the pupillary area. The pupillary area is cleared of vitreous and the presence of any strand is confirmed with the use of triamcinolone acetonide 0.5 cc injection. A 3-piece foldable IOL is injected beneath the nuclear fragment in a way that the leading haptic is guided and placed above the capsulorhexis while the trailing haptic is left extruded at the corneal incision (Figs 3.22A and B). The phacoemulsification probe is introduced into the eye and the nuclear fragments are emulsified (Figs 3.22C and D). Using a dialer in the non-dominant hand, the surgeon maneuvers the optic-haptic junction on the trailing haptic side so that the IOL blocks the pupil. Keeping the trailing haptic outside the incision enables adjustment of the IOL position in case if the nucleus rotates thus reducing the risk of IOL drop. Any residual cortex is then removed using the vitrectomy probe in suction mode with low aspiration. The IOL is maneuvered over the capsular remnants in the ciliary sulcus (Figs 3.22E and F). If the capsular support is inadequate, a glued IOL procedure is performed. The infusion cannula/anterior chamber maintainer is removed, and the trailing haptic is then dialed into position above the capsulorhexis and the stability of the IOL checked. The incisions are hydrated and checked for stability.

GLUED IOL SCAFFOLD

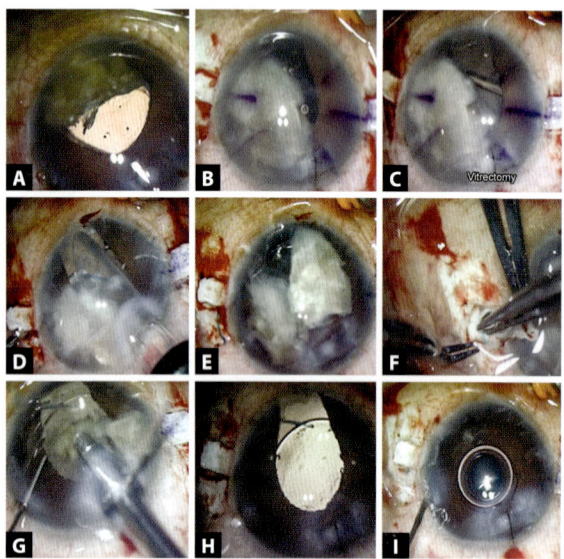

Figs 3.23A to I Glued IOL scaffold. (A) Following a posterior capsule rupture, the nuclear fragment is levitated into the anterior chamber; (B) Two partial thickness scleral flaps are made 180° opposite to each other; (C) Sclerotomy port created with a 20 G needle as in a glued IOL surgery and vitrectomy is being done; (D) Corneal tunnel is framed and a 3-piece foldable IOL is injected beneath the nuclear fragments; (E) Both the haptics are externalized; (F) Haptics are tucked into the scleral pockets created with a 26 G needle; (G) Phaco probe is introduced and the nuclear pieces are being emulsified; (H) All the nuclear fragments are emulsified; (I) Stromal hydration is done and the corneal wound is closed with 10-0 suture. Fibrin glue is applied beneath the scleral flaps and the conjunctiva

In cases of intraoperative PCR, the phacoemulsification procedure is withheld. The remaining nuclear pieces are brought in to the anterior chamber (Fig. 3.23A). An infusion cannula is fixed and scleral flaps are fashioned as in glued IOL surgery (Fig. 3.23B). Sclerotomy is then created with a 20-gauge needle approximately 1 mm behind the limbus under the scleral flaps. A 23 g vitrectomy probe is passed through the sclerotomy to perform vitrectomy so that all the tractional forces in the vitreous are nullified (Fig. 3.23C). Vitrectomy is an essential step in the surgery as one can otherwise land up with a retinal detachment postoperatively.

The three-piece foldable IOL is loaded onto the injector and the cartridge passed into the anterior chamber (AC) (Fig. 3.23D). The haptic tip should be slightly out of the cartridge so that when one goes to grasp the haptic with the glued IOL forceps it is easy. The haptic tip is grasped with the glued IOL forceps and while the IOL is unfolded the haptic tip is still caught. The chances of the IOL falling down are not there as the haptic is caught with the forceps and the trailing haptic is still outside the clear corneal incision. Using the handshake technique the trailing haptic is externalized (Fig. 3.23E). If the nuclear pieces are occupying a lot of space in the AC this maneuver is sometimes difficult. One should use viscoelastic to dislodge the pieces to the side to gain visualization.

A 26 G needle is used to create the Scharioth pocket and the haptics are tucked into the intrascleral pocket (Fig. 3.23 F).

Phacoemulsification of the nuclear pieces is then performed (Fig. 3.23G) as an artificial posterior capsule has been created using the combination of the glued IOL and the IOL scaffold technique (Fig. 3.23H). This prevents the nuclear fragments from falling into the vitreous cavity. Finally air is injected into the AC and fibrin glue is used to seal the scleral flaps (Fig. 3.23I).

PRE-DESCEMET'S ENDOTHELIAL KERATYOPLASTY WITH GLUED IOL

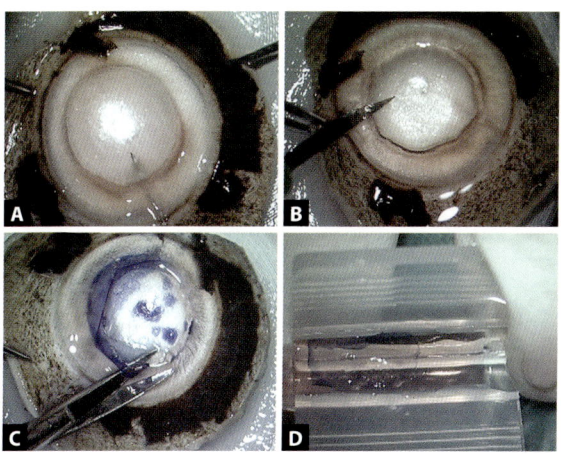

Figs 3.24A to D Donor graft preparation in pre-Descemet's endothelial keratoplasty (PDEK). (A) With the endothelial side up, a 30 G needle attached to a 5 mL syringe is introduced from the periphery and air is injected so as to create a Type-1 bubble that characteristically spreads from center to periphery; (B) The edge of the bb is penetrated with a side-port blade; (C) Trypan blue is injected inside the bubble so as to stain the graft. The graft is then cut along its peripheral edge and is harvested; (D) The graft is loaded on to the injector of a foldable IOL

Early evidence to support the existence of a distinct pre-Descemet's layer (Dua's layer) of tissue was presented by Harminder Dua in 2007 and followed by a detailed paper

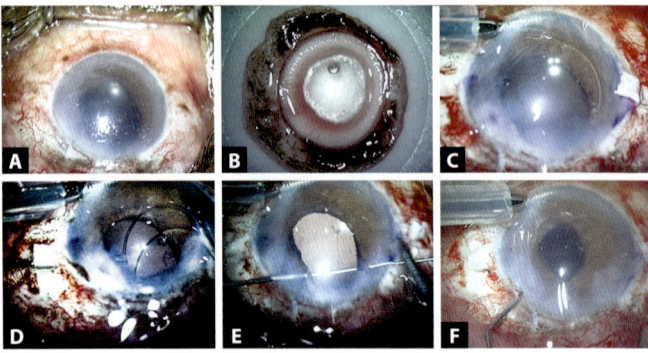

Figs 3.25A to F It takes two to tango—Pre-Descemet's endothelial keratoplasty (PDEK) with glued IOL. (A) Pre-operative photograph of the cornea of the patient with pseudophakic bullous keratopathy. PC IOL in AC; (B) A type-1 big bubble (bb) between the pre-Descemet's layer (Dua's layer) and stroma is formed. Note the bb does not reach the periphery of the cornea as there are firm adhesions between the pre-Descemet's layer and stroma in the periphery. If a bubble is created that extends to the corneoscleral limbus it is a type-2 (pre-Descemet's) bb that symbolizes that the air has formed between the Descemet's membrane and the Pre-Descemet's layer; (C) AC maintainer is fixed and sclera flaps created; (D) Glued IOL surgery is performed and haptics are externalized; (E) Pupilloplasty; (F) Pupilloplasty completed with glued IOL in place. Eye is now ready for PDEK surgery

wherein evidence is presented to further support the presence of the distinct pre-Descemet's layer. Addition of a 10 micron (mean value) of this pre-Descemet's layer to the endothelial graft can be exploited in generating tissue for endothelial transplant,

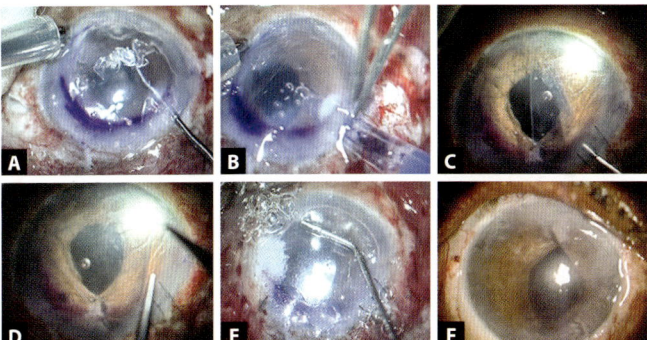

Figs 3.26A to F It takes two to tango—Pre-Descemet's endothelial keratoplasty with glued IOL. (A) Descematorhexis being performed; (B) The PDEK graft is injected into the anterior chamber with the help of the injector; (C) Graft is subsequently unrolled with air and fluidics. An endoilluminator is used to help in ascertaining orientation and checking the unrolling of the graft (E-PDEK); (D) The graft is unrolled after checking correct orientation; (E) Air is injected under the graft to appose it to the cornea. PDEK graft is attached to the cornea with a complete air fill of the anterior chamber. Then glue applied to the scleral flaps; (F) Postoperative one week image of the patient

allowing easier handling and insertion of the tissue as it does not tend to scroll as much as the DM, with the pre-descemets layer splinting the DM. Pre-Descemet's endothelial keratoplasty (PDEK) is the term we have given to describe a technique in which the donor endothelial-DM complex with the additional pre-Descemet's layer is transplanted. This technique was started by Amar Agarwal and Harminder Dua.

SURGICAL CONSIDERATIONS FOR COMBINED PROCEDURE

The main advantage of combining PDEK and Glued IOL surgery is patient convenience. Patients undergo only one surgery, attend fewer appointments, and deal with only one set of postoperative medications.

Although a combined surgical procedure is not significantly more complex than PDEK surgery alone, a few concerns must be addressed, especially for novice surgeons. During the surgery, the surgeon must be prepared for a decreased view secondary to guttata or haze, decreased anterior chamber stability (in cases requiring explantation of a previous IOL), increased chances of graft dislocation (intraoperative miosis is often required), increased intraocular inflammation that may lead to increased endothelial cell damage, and a potential risk of problems with the anterior chamber air fill due to air diversion into the vitreous.

SURGICAL TECHNIQUE

The initial step involves successful harvesting of the donor lenticule followed by Glued IOL procedure (minus the application of glue to seal the scleral flaps) followed by recipient bed preparation and donor lenticule insertion. Application of fibrin glue to seal the scleral flaps is then ensued so as to ensure that it is not washed off by the fluids emanating and egressing from the eye.

Step 1: Donor Graft Preparation (Figs 3.24A to D)

In this an air filled 5 mL syringe with an attached 30 G needle is introduced from the corneoscleral disc with bevel up till the center of the donor lenticule with the endothelial side up (Fig. 3.24A). As air is injected, a Type 1 bubble is formed with a distinct edge all around. The edge of the bubble at extreme periphery is perforated (Fig. 3.24B) followed by injection of trypan blue into the bubble to stain the graft, which is then cut all around the trephine mark with corneo-scleral scissors (Fig. 3.24C). The graft is then stored in the storage media and loaded onto a cartridge of a foldable IOL injector (Fig. 3.24D).

Step 2: Glued IOL Technique (Figs 3.25 to 3.27)

This consists of making two partial scleral thickness flaps approximately 2.5 by 2.5 mm in size and 180° opposite to each other. The epithelium of the recipient eye is often debrided due to epithelium decompensation which hinders the intraoperative view to a great extent. An anterior chamber (AC) maintainer is introduced in the lower quadrant and a sclerotomy wound is created with a 20 G needle approximately 1 mm away from limbus beneath the scleral flaps and the entire glued IOL surgery is performed till the tucking of the haptics in the scleral pockets (Figs 3.25A to F). AC maintainer helps to maintain the AC through out the surgery and the use of viscoelastic is deterred as it is important not to leave residual viscoelastic in the anterior chamber as it is thought to potentially hamper good adhesion between the donor corneal disk and the recipient corneal stroma.

142 | Phacoemulsification

PREOPERATIVE AND POSTOPERATIVE IMAGE OF PATIENT OF PDEK WITH GLUED IOL

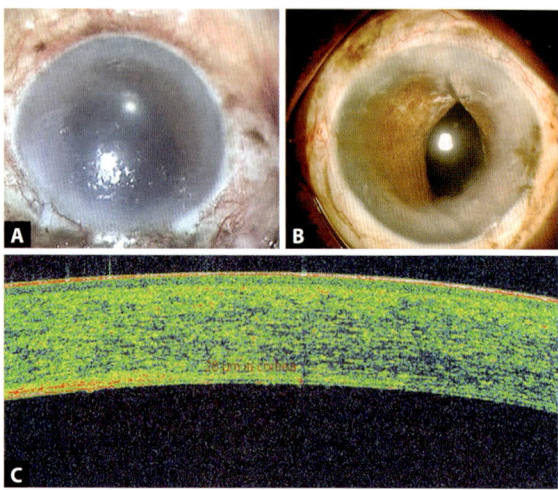

Figs 3.27A to C It takes two to tango—Pre-Descemet's endothelial keratoplasty with glued IOL. (A) Preoperative case of pseudophakic bullous keratopathy with a PC IOL placed in the AC; (B) Postoperative- 7 month 20/30 vision; (C) Anterior segment OCT showing the graft attached

Step 3

The recipient cornea is marked with a trephine so as to outline the area of DM to be excised. A reverse sinskey hook is introduced into the anterior chamber and descematorrhexis is performed corresponding to the margins of the epithelial mark (Fig. 3.26A).

The DM is then stripped off and is removed from the anterior chamber. The donor pre-Descemet's roll is loaded on to the cartridge of a foldable IOL injector and the spring of the injector is removed (as originally improvised by Francis Price) so as to prevent any damage to the donor graft (Fig. 3.26B). The donor roll is injected into the anterior chamber and the graft is slowly unfolded with air and fluidics avoiding any direct contact with the graft so as to minimize the trauma (Figs 3.26C and D). The PDEK graft rolls like a DMEK graft with the endothelium on the outer side, although due to the splinting effect of PDL the rolling of tissue graft is comparatively less. After proper orientation of the graft, air is injected beneath it to facilitate proper adhesion to the posterior corneal stroma (Figs 3.26E and F). About 30 minutes is allowed to elapse to facilitate initial donor recipient corneal disk adherence. Postoperatively, the patient is asked to lay flat in the recovery room for about an hour and also to lay flat for the most part during the first post-operative day.

After surgery, all patients undergo pressure patching and supine positioning overnight. Beginning the next morning, 0.1% dexamethasone sodium phosphate and moxifloxacin eye drops are administered every 2 hourly for 1 week and the every 4 hourly for next 3 weeks. Topical steroid drops are then tapered to 3 times daily in the second month, twice daily in the third month, and once daily from the fourth month onward. The postoperative photograph of the patient taken at 7 months follow-up shows a well centered graft and a clear cornea that is confirmed on OCT (Figs 3.27 A to C).

REFRACTIVE CONCERN

Performing IOL implantation before a corneal procedure involves lot of refractive instability and unpredictable keratometry values; therefore, predicting the lens implant power before a corneal procedure can present challenges. Studies of lens power calculations associated with keratoplasty have shown that an effective way of reducing postoperative ametropia is to perform keratoplasty first, followed by lens extraction and IOL implantation at a later date. Flowers et al. reported 95% of patients within ±2.00 D of intended postoperative target refraction following PKP and cataract extraction with IOL placement performed secondarily.

SECTION 4

Microincision Cataract Surgery
(Phakonit and Microphakonit)

Amar Agarwal
Priya Narang

CLEAR CORNEAL INCISION MADE WITH A SPECIAL KNIFE (MST, USA)

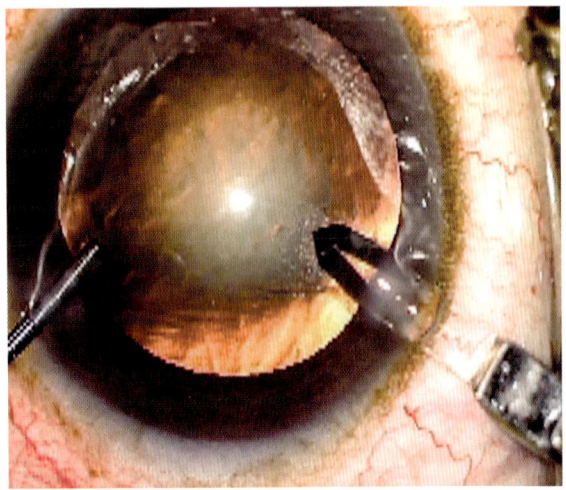

Fig. 4.1 Clear corneal incision framed with a special keratome designed by MST, USA. The globe stabilization rod helps to stabilize the eye during the surgery. Note the left hand has a globe stabilization rod to stabilize the eye. (Geuder, germany). This knife can frame an incision from sub 1 mm to 1.2 mm

On 15th August 1998, the author (Amar Agarwal) performed the first 1 mm cataract surgery by **PHAKONIT** technique. The term '**PHAKONIT**' designates phaco (PHAKO) being done with a needle (N) opening via an incision (I) and with the phako tip

Microincision Cataract Surgery (Phakonit and Microphakonit)

(T). It is also known as Phako being done with a Needle Incision Technology. In this the cataract was removed through a bimanual phaco technique and it was performed without any anesthesia. The first live surgery in the world of Phakonit was performed on August 22nd 1998 at Pune, India by the author (Amar Agarwal) at the Phaco and Refractive surgery conference.

The point of concern with this technique was to find an IOL, which would pass through such a small incision. Eventually on 2nd October 2001 the author (Amar Agarwal) performed a case of Phakonit with the implantation of a Rollable IOL. The lens used was a special lens from ThinOptx that worked on Fresnel principle and was designed by Wayne Callahan from USA. The first such ultrathin lens was implanted by Jairo Hoyos from Spain that was later modified by the author (Amar Agarwal) into a special 5 mm optic rollable IOL.

A 26 G needle attached to a 1 mL syringe filled with viscoelastic is taken and pierced in the eye in the area where the side port incision has to be framed. The viscoelastic is then injected inside the eye. This distends the eye so that the clear corneal incision can be made. A special knife can be used for this purpose. Note in the Figure 4.1 the left hand holds a globe stabilization rod (Geuder, Germany). This helps to stabilize the eye while creating the clear corneal incision. The special knife is held in the dominant hand and it helps to create an incision of either sub 1 mm or 1.2 mm depending on the diameter of the knife chosen by the surgeon. If the surgeon choses a sub 1 mm knife then a 21 gauge irrigating chopper and a 0.8 mm phaco needle is the preferred choice.

CAPSULORHEXIS INITIATED WITH A NEEDLE

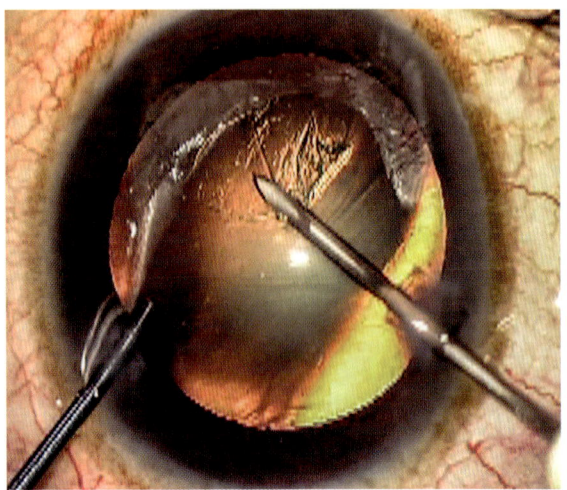

Fig. 4.2 Capsulorhexis initiated with a needle

Capsulorhexis is performed either with a 26 G needle (Fig. 4.2) or with a capsulorhexis forceps through the corneal incision and the choice depends entirely on the surgeon's preference. In pediatric and young patients it is preferable to do rhexis with a forceps as it offers better control over the edges of the flap created. In young patients, the surgeon should intend to create a rhexis of around 5 mm initially as it often tends to run in the periphery due to increased posterior pressure and elasticity of the capsule.

While performing the rhexis, it is important to start the rhexis from the center and move the needle to the right and then downward. This is important, as the concepts have changed and it is better to remember it as superior, inferior, right or left. If the surgeon happens to start the rhexis from the center and move towards the left then the weakest point of the rhexis is generally where it ends. In other words, the point where the surgeon tends to lose the rhexis is near its completion. So the surgeon will have an incomplete rhexis on the left-hand side either inferiorly or superiorly. As, the phaco probe is always moved down and to the left so with every stroke of movement with the phaco probe the rhexis gets extended posteriorly creating a posterior capsular rupture. Alternatively, if the surgeon performs the rhexis from the center and move to the right and pushes the flap inferiorly then in a case of incomplete rhexis it will be near the end of the rhexis and it will be located superiorly and to the right. Any incomplete rhexis can extend and create a posterior capsular tear but in the latter scenario, the chances of survival are better. This is because we are moving the phaco probe down and to the left, but the rhexis is incomplete up and to the right.

MST RHEXIS FORCEPS USED TO PERFORM THE RHEXIS IN A MATURE CATARACT

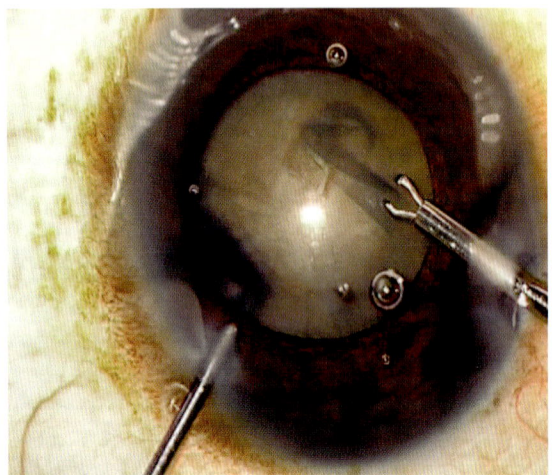

Fig. 4.3 MST capsulorhexis forceps used to perform the capsulorhexis in a mature cataract. Trypan blue stains the anterior capsule for better visualization. Note the trypan blue staining the anterior capsule

In the left hand a straight rod is held to stabilize the eye. This is known as the Globe stabilization rod. The advantage of this is that the movements of the eye can be controlled as the surgeon performs either a 'Topical' or a 'No anesthesia' cataract surgery. Microsurgical Technology (USA) has designed an excellent capsulorhexis forceps for Phakonit (Fig. 4.3) that passes through a 1 mm incision. Surgeons comfortable with a forceps can use this special forceps during Phakonit surgery.

DESIGNS OF AGARWAL IRRIGATING CHOPPERS

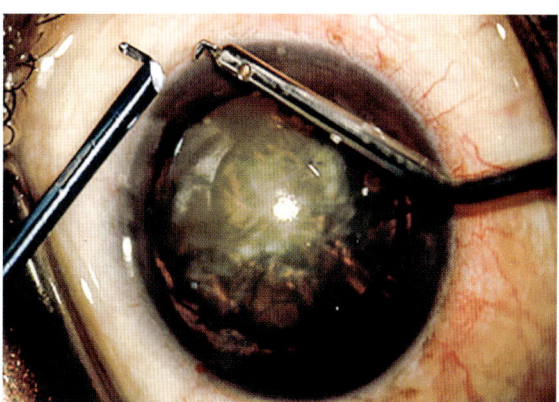

Fig. 4.4 Designs of Agarwal irrigating choppers. The one on the left has an end opening for fluid (microsurgical technology). The one on the right has openings on the either sides (Geuder–Germany)

Two designs of irrigating choppers that are designed are designated in the picture. On the left is the 'Agarwal irrigating chopper' made by the MST (Microsurgical Technology) company that is incorporated in the Duet system (Fig. 4.4). The irrigating chopper on the right is made by Geuder, Germany.

Notice in the right figure the opening for the fluid is end opening, whereas the one on the left the chopper has two openings on the sides. Depending on the convenience of the surgeon, the surgeon can decide upon the design of irrigating chopper to be used.

PHAKONIT IRRIGATING CHOPPER AND PHAKO PROBE WITHOUT THE SLEEVE INSIDE THE EYE

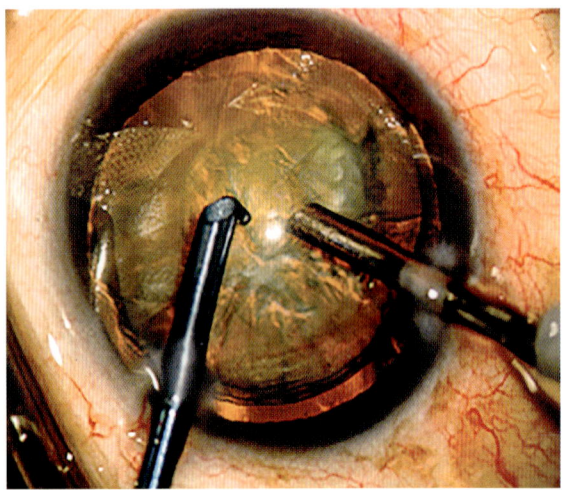

Fig. 4.5 Phakonit irrigating chopper and phaco probe without the sleeve inside the eye

The procedure of Phakonit (Fig. 4.5) can be performed with any phaco machine. The usual parameters set are:

Power-50% phaco power: Start in the continuous mode and once chopping has been done then shift to the pulse mode.

Suction-100 mm of Hg: The surgeon should use an air pump or an antichamber collapser to eliminate surge.

Flow rate: 20–24 mL/min.

Phaco needle: If the surgeon uses a 0.8 mm phaco needle with a 21 gauge irrigating chopper then sub 1 mm cataract surgery is eventually achieved.

Continuous irrigation over corneal incision is preferred as it negates the possibility of a corneal burn.

PHAKONIT BEING DONE

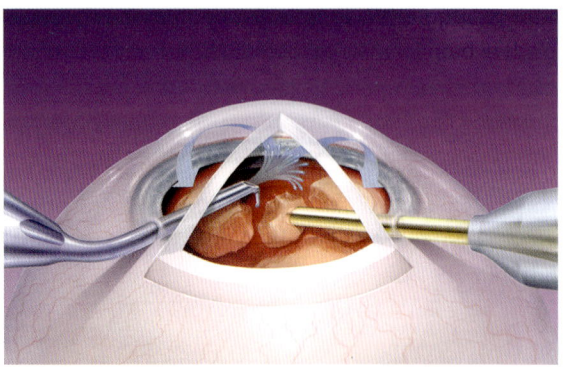

Fig. 4.6 Phakonit being performed. Notice the irrigating chopper with an end opening
(*Courtesy:* Larry Laks, MST, USA)

This is a specially designed irrigating chopper (Fig. 4.6) to facilitate the procedure of 'Phakonit'.

BIMANUAL IRRIGATION ASPIRATION COMPLETED

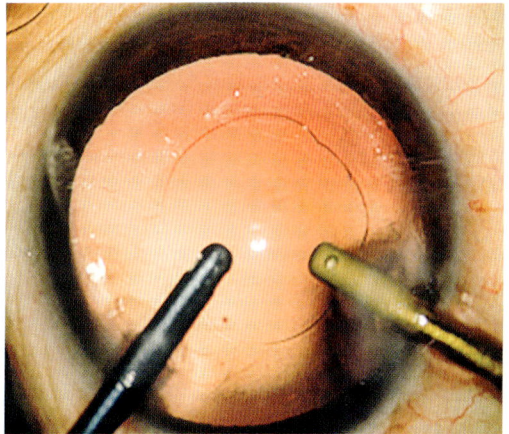

Fig. 4.7 Irrigation aspiration completed. Cortical wash-up done with the bimanual irrigation aspiration technique

Following irrigation-aspiration (Fig. 4.7), the surgeon can inject vancomycin inside the eye at the end of the surgery to prevent endophthalmitis. For this the intraoperative protocol is:
- 250 mg vial of vancomycin is taken to be dissolved in 25 mL of Ringer lactate (RL) or balanced salt solution (BSS)
- This will give a concentration of 1 mg in 0.1 mL
- At the end of the surgery, insert 0.1 mL of vancomycin containing 1 mg into the capsular bag behind the IOL. If need be additional BSS/RL can be injected into the eye to make the eye firm.

SOFT TIP IRRIGATION-ASPIRATION FROM MST, USA

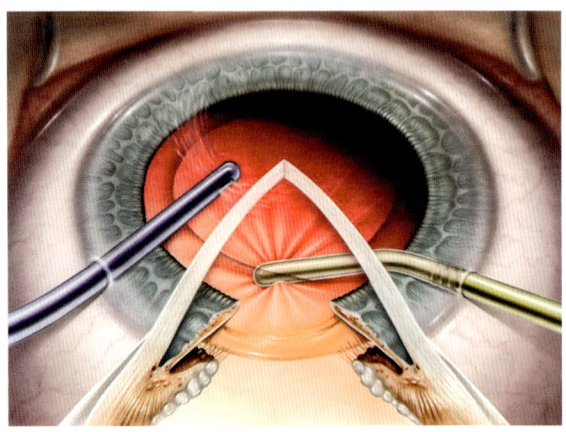

Fig. 4.8 Soft tip irrigation aspiration
(*Courtesy:* Larry Laks-MST)

Microsurgical Technology (USA) has designed a soft tip I/A (Fig. 4.8) that is very safe for the posterior capsule.

THINOPTX ROLLER CUM INJECTOR INSERTING THE IOL IN THE CAPSULAR BAG

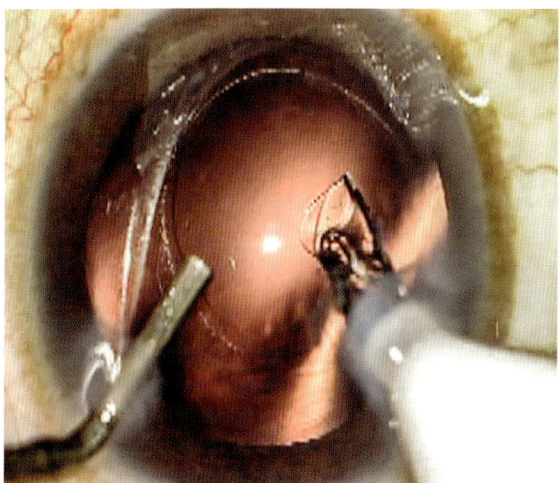

Fig. 4.9 ThinOptx roller cum injector inserting the IOL in the capsular bag

ThinOptx have made a special injector that not only rolls the lens but also inserts the lens (Fig. 4.9). This avoids the need to use our fingers for rolling the lens. In the figure a special injector injecting the IOL in the capsular bag is noticed. The tip of the nozzle is kept at the edge of the incision.

COMPARISON BETWEEN PHACO FOLDABLE IOL AND PHAKONIT THINOPTX IOL

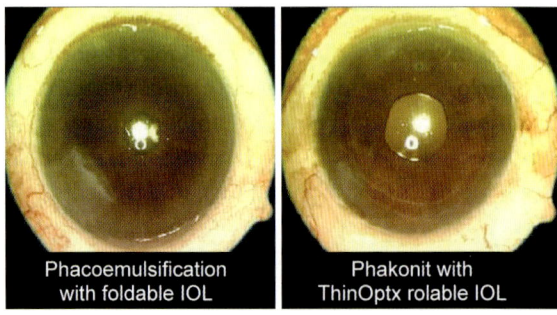

Fig. 4.10 An illustrative photograph showing the comparison between phaco foldable IOL and phakonit ThinOptx IOL. The figure on the left shows a case of phako with a foldable iol and the figure on the right shows phakonit with a ThinOptx rollable IOL

ThinOptx the company that manufactures these lenses has patented technology that allows the manufacture of lenses with plus or minus 30 diopters of correction on the thickness of 100 microns. The ThinOptx technology developed by Wayne Callahan, Scott Callahan and Joe Callahan is not limited to material choice, but is achieved instead of an evolutionary optic and unprecedented nano-scale manufacturing process. The lens is made from off-the-shelf hydrophilic material, which is similar to several IOL materials already on the market (Fig. 4.10). The key to the ThinOptx lens is the optic design and nano-precision manufacturing. The basic advantage of this lens is that they are Ultra-Thin lenses. One of the authors (Amar Agarwal) modified this lens to make a special 5 mm optic rollable IOL.

The Acrylic IOL is manufactured by the AcriTec company in Berlin, Germany. This lens is a sterile foldable intraocular lens made of hydrophobic acrylate. The intraocular lens consists of highly purified biocompatible hydrophobic acrylate with chemically bonded UV-absorber. It is a single piece foldable IOL like a plate-haptic IOL. The lens is sterilized by autoclaving. The lens comes in a sterile vial, filled with water and wrapped in a sterile pouch.

MICROPHAKONIT

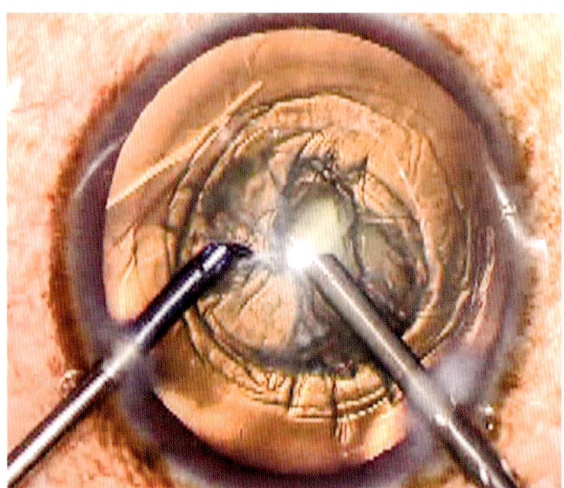

Fig. 4.11 In microphakonit, 0.7 mm irrigating chopper and 0.7 mm phaco tip without the sleeve is seen inside the eye. The assistant continuously irrigates the phaco probe area to prevent corneal burns

On May 21st 2005, for the first time a 0.7 mm phaco needle tip with a 0.7 mm irrigating chopper was used by the authors (Am A) to remove cataracts through the smallest incision possible as of now. This is called microphakonit (Fig. 4.11).

Lary Laks from MST, made a special 0.7 mm phaco needle for microphakonit.

The inner diameter of the phaco tip regulates the flow rate/perceived efficiency. In order to increase the allowed aspiration flow rate from what a standard 0.7 mm tip would be, MST (Larry Laks) made the walls thinner, thus increasing the inner diameter. This would facilitate better speed at low diameter. With the utilization of gas forced infusion the system would work very well.

MICROPHAKONIT COMPLETED. THE NUCLEUS HAS BEEN REMOVED

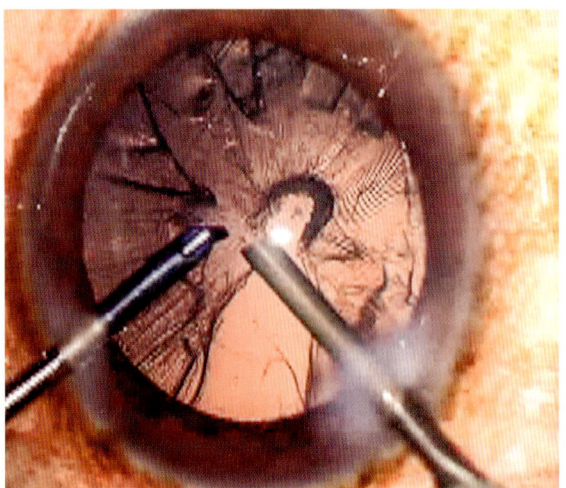

Fig. 4.12 Microphakonit is completed and the nucleus is completely emulsified

An end-opening irrigating chopper is preferred as the bore of the irrigating chopper is smaller (Fig. 4.12) and the amount of fluid effusing out of it would be less and so an end-opening chopper would maintain the fluidics better. With the additional back up of gas forced infusion, the amount of fluid entering and exiting into the anterior chamber can be balanced.

The problem encountered in phakonit was the destabilization of the anterior chamber during surgery. It was solved to a certain extent by using an 18-gauge irrigating chopper. Eventually, Dr Sunita Agarwal suggested the use of an antichamber collapser, which injects air into the infusion bottle. This pushes more fluid into the eye through the irrigating chopper and also prevents surge.

BIMANUAL IRRIGATION-ASPIRATION WITH THE 0.7 mm SET

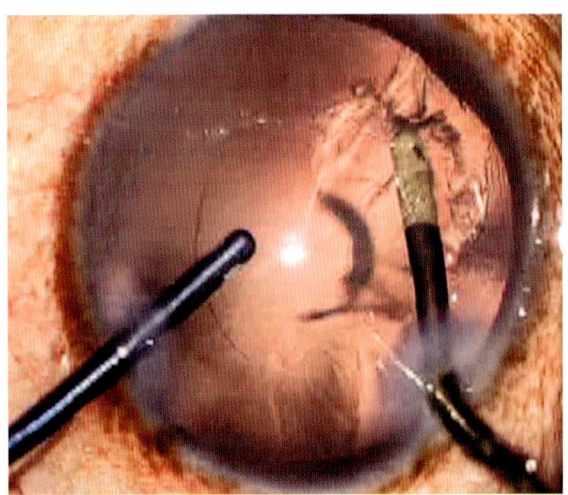

Fig. 4.13 Bimanual irrigation-aspiration with 0.7 mm set

Bimanual irrigation-aspiration is done with the bimanual irrigation-aspiration instruments (Fig. 4.13) designed by Microsurgical Technology (USA). The previous set we used was the 0.9 mm set. With microphakonit it is necessary to use a 0.7 mm bimanual I/A set so that after the nucleus removal there is no need to enlarge the incision.

BIMANUAL IRRIGATION-ASPIRATION COMPLETED

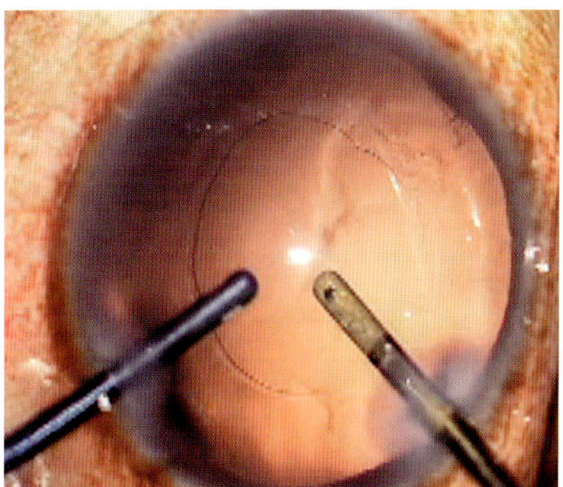

Fig. 4.14 Bimanual irrigation-aspiration is completed

With microphakonit a 0.7 mm set is used for the cataract. At present this is the smallest size available for a cataract surgery (Fig. 4.14). With further evolution over a period of time, better instruments and designs can be achieved.

Index

Page numbers followed by *f* refer to figure

A

Acetazolamide 120
Agarwal irrigating choppers, designs of 151, 151*f*
Anoxia theory 110
Anterior segment examination 114
Antimicrobial therapy 100
Aqueous biotoxic complex 110

B

Balanced salt solution 2
Bimanual cortical aspiration 20, 20*f*
Bimanual irrigation aspiration 155, 155*f*, 164, 165, 165*f*
Boston keratoprosthesis 129

C

Candida parapsilosis 94
Capillary leakage 115
Capsular tension rings 70
Capsulorhexis 11, 11*f*-12*f*, 148*f*
    flap 12
Centrifuge method 91
Charged coupled device 61
Chopping nuclear hemisegments 17
Cionni's capsular tension ring 39, 39*f*
Complete petaloid ring 115
Corticosteroid therapy 103
Crystalline lens, anterior dislocation of 123*f*
Cystoid macular edema 107, 107*f*, 108, 116
Cysts of CME, origin of 111

D

Dislocated capsular bag IOL complex 131*f*
Dislocated IOL on retina 72

E

Endophthalmitis 90, 90*f*, 99, 99*f*, 101
    acute postoperative 93
    chronic bacterial 94
    vitrectomy study 92
Extracapsular cataract extraction 94
Extracellular theory 111

F

Flower petal appearance 107*f*
Fluorescein angiography 107*f*
Fundus fluorescein angiography 114

G

Glued intrascleral fixation 42
Glued IOL 123, 125
 procedure 125*f*
 scaffold 134*f*
 technique 141

H

Handshake technique 125*f*
Henle, nerve fiber layer of 108
Hyperbaric oxygen 119
Hypermature cataract 38

I

Incision, plane of 10
Indocyanine green 33
Inflammation theory 109
Internal gas forced infusion 4*f*
Intracellular theory 111
Intraocular lens 91
Intraocular pressure 4

Intravitreal antimicrobial therapy 102
IOL scaffold 132*f*
Iridodialysis repair 127*f*
Iris coloboma 43, 43*f*
Irrigation aspiration 155*f*

L

Lens
 coloboma with glued IOL, management of 69
 subluxation of 37, 37*f*
Lenticular coloboma 41, 69*f*

M

Macular edema 108
Marfan's syndrome 38, 41, 42
Massive lens coloboma, management of 69*f*
Massive lenticular coloboma 41*f*
Massive traumatic iridodialysis 127*f*
Microincision cataract surgery 9, 145
Microphakonit 160, 160*f*, 162*f*
Morganella morganii 93
Müller's cells 117

N

Nd-YAG laser vitreolysis 120

O

Ophthalmic endoscopic system, principle of 60, 60*f*
Ophthalmoscopy, indirect 114
Optical coherence tomography 116
Oral NSAID therapy 119

P

Pars plana vitrectomy 132*f*
Partial petaloid ring 115
Perfluorocarbon liquids 76, 77
  types of 76
Perifoveal edema
  minimal 115
  moderate 115
Peripheral annular Soemmering ring 44*f*
Phaco foldable IOL 158, 158*f*
Phaco needle 153
Phakonit irrigating chopper 152, 152*f*
Phakonit technique 146
Phakonit ThinOptx IOL 158, 158*f*
Polar cataract, posterior 30
Pre-Descemet's
  endothelial keratoplasty 137*f*-139*f*, 142*f*
  layer of tissue 137, 138
Propionibacterium acnes 94
  endophthalmitis 94
Pseudoexfoliation syndrome 24, 25*f*, 38
Pseudophakic bullous keratopathy 138*f*, 142*f*
Pseudophakic CME with
  ACIOL 121
  PCIOL 122

R

Ringer lactate 155

S

Severe perifoveal edema 115
Sieper's technique, modified 43*f*
Sleeveless extrusion cannula assisted levitation of dropped IOL 72*f*
Sleeveless phacotip assisted levitation of dropped nucleus technique 50, 50*f*, 53
Soemmering ring 44
Soft tip irrigation aspiration 156, 156*f*
Staphylococcus aureus 93
Staphylococcus epidermidis 94
Suction filter method 90
Synechia 28, 28*f*

Systemic antimicrobial therapy 102
Systemic steroids 119

T

Temporary haptic externalization 80, 80*f*
Topical NSAIDs 119
Traumatic iridodialysis 127
Typical fish tail sign 46

V

Vertical chop 15
Vitrectomy 56, 104
  techniques 105
Vitreous traction theory 109

Z

Zonular fibers 37*f*